DR ANNE TOWNSEND

The Great Body Book

THE INSIDE GUIDE TO WHAT MAKES YOU SPECIAL

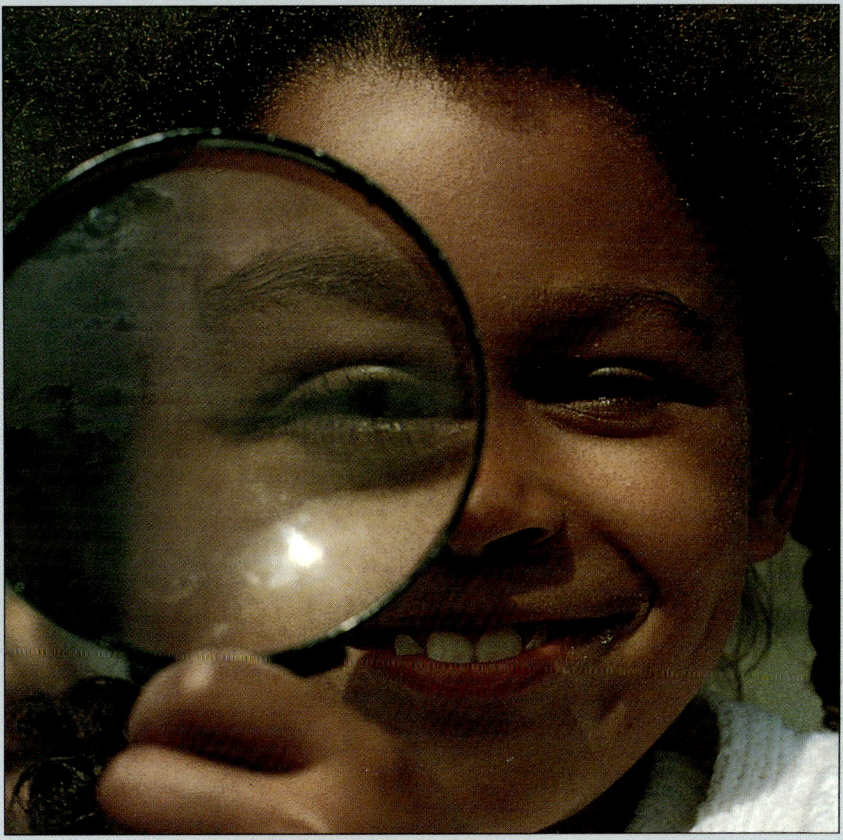

A LION BOOK

Published by
Lion Publishing plc
Sandy Lane West, Oxford, England
ISBN 0 7459 2755 6
Albatross Books Pty Ltd
PO Box 320, Sutherland, NSW 2232, Australia
ISBN 0 7324 0882 2

First edition 1984
Reprinted 1985, 1986, 1987, 1990
Second edition 1994

Acknowledgments
Medical adviser to this new edition: Dr Penny Moore

Photographs
David Alexander: spread 14
Lion Publishing: title page, spreads 1 (top left, lower left and bottom left), 2 (bottom right), 10 (top right), 12 (top right), 15 (top right), 19 (small picture), 20 (right page centre right and bottom)
Oxford Scientific Films: spreads 2 (top right), 13 (left)
Steve Rock: spreads 1 (upper left), 6 (right), 11 (both), 12 (top right corner), 13 (right)
Nicholas Rous: spread 20 (right page top right)
Science Photo Library: spread 3 (right)
Skjold Photography: spreads 5, 20 (right page top left and centre left)
John Williams: spreads 9 (far right), 15 (bottom right), 16, 17, 20 (left)
ZEFA: spreads 1 (right), 6 (left), 7 (both), 8, 9 (bottom right), 10 (top left and bottom right), 18, 19 (main picture)

Illustrations
Cartoons by Kim Blundell
Diagrams by Oxford Illustrators

A catalogue record for this book is available from the British Library

Printed and bound in Malaysia

CONTENTS

IT'S AMAZING!

The way the human body works is amazing. There are so many questions to ask about it. What happens to the food we eat? How do people go on breathing when they're asleep? How does bleeding stop? Why doesn't it hurt to have your hair cut? Why do some cuts heal well and others leave a scar?

It's taken years and years for scientists to find out the answers to these questions—and many more besides. Amazingly, there's a lot that scientists have still to find out! Reading this book is a good way to start finding out for yourself how your body works, and what make you the special person you are

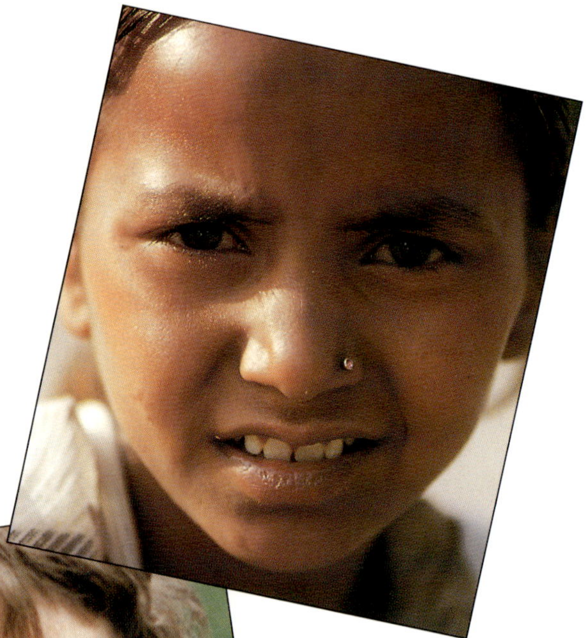

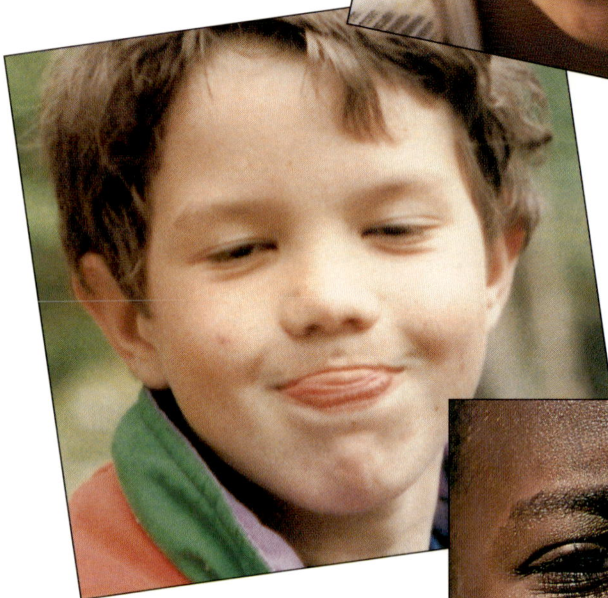

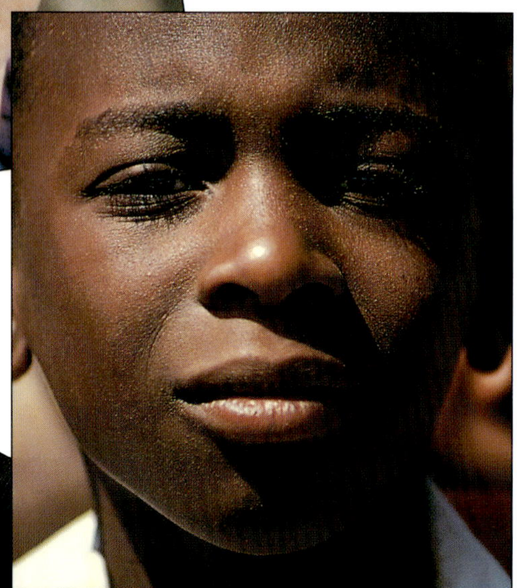

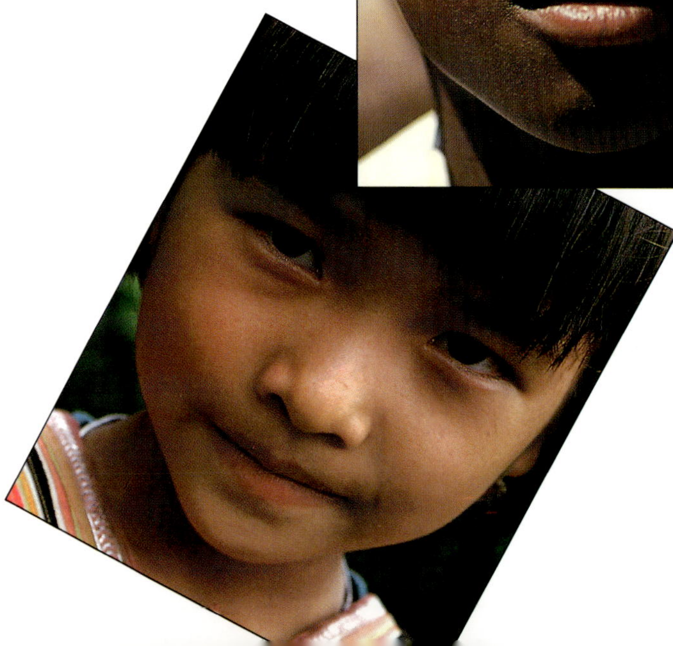

BODYWORKS

It's easy to see the outside of someone's body. A person has arms and legs, feet and hands, a body and a head. The skin is smooth, with hair in places—most especially on the top of the head!

Inside, under the skin, is a miraculous inner world that never stops working until the person dies. Organs such as lungs and a heart are hard at work. Nerves and blood vessels, muscles and bones connect everything together.

In a healthy body, all the different parts work together, doing what they're supposed to do in the right way and at the right time. It's a design masterpiece!

EVERY ONE UNIQUE!

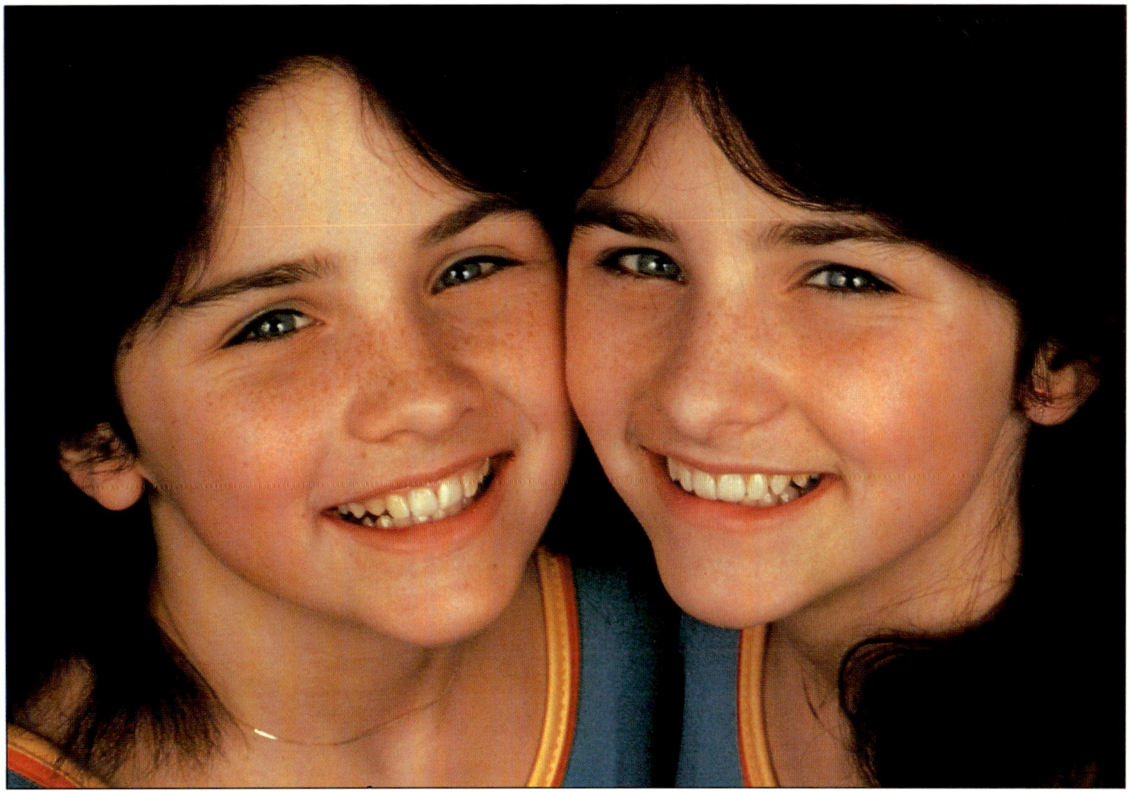

Human bodies all follow the same amazing design. But there are lots and lots of variations! Unless you are one of identical twins, you won't find anyone in the whole world who looks exactly like you.

Even so-called identical twins are not exactly the same. Look closely at the finger nearest your thumb—your index finger. On the pad of that finger you can see tiny grooves and ridges in a pattern. This pattern is your fingerprint. No one in the whole world has the same fingerprint as you.

Each person is special in other ways too: in the kind of person they are, in the things they enjoy doing, in the way they laugh . . . and everything else about them.

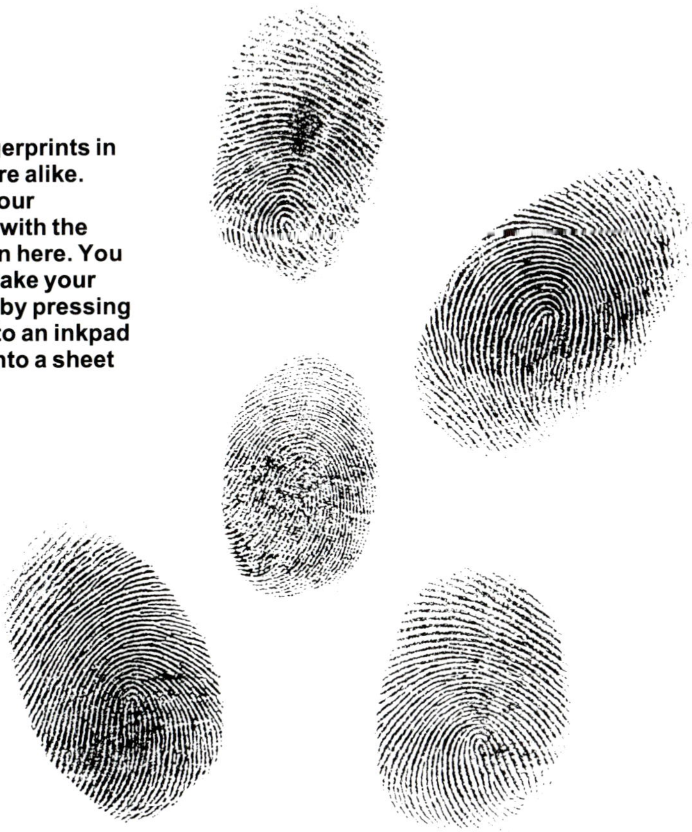

No two fingerprints in the world are alike. Compare your fingerprint with the ones shown here. You can easily take your fingerprint by pressing a finger onto an inkpad and then onto a sheet of paper.

WHY ME?

Scientists are very good at finding out answers to some types of questions: questions about *what* bodies are made of, and *how* they work. But *why* are there people at all? Why you? Why me?

Science isn't very good at answering *why* questions. But throughout the ages people have told stories that try to explain why the world exists, and what the point of being alive really is.

One of these stories is found in the first book of the Bible—a book that is special to Jews and to Christians. It says that in the beginning, God made the world and everything in it. And God made people to enjoy the world and to look after it.

THE BODY'S BUILDING BLOCKS—CELLS

A building is made up of many different parts: it may have thousands of bricks to make the walls, and several strong beams to support the ceiling. And the human body is made up of many millions of different parts. They are called cells.

There are so many cells that it would be impossible for anyone to try to count them. Cells are so small that you can only see them with a microscope.

All the cells in your body are made in the same basic pattern, but they have different shapes and designs depending on the type of work they have to do.

A cell is very, very small. But every cell has at least three parts:

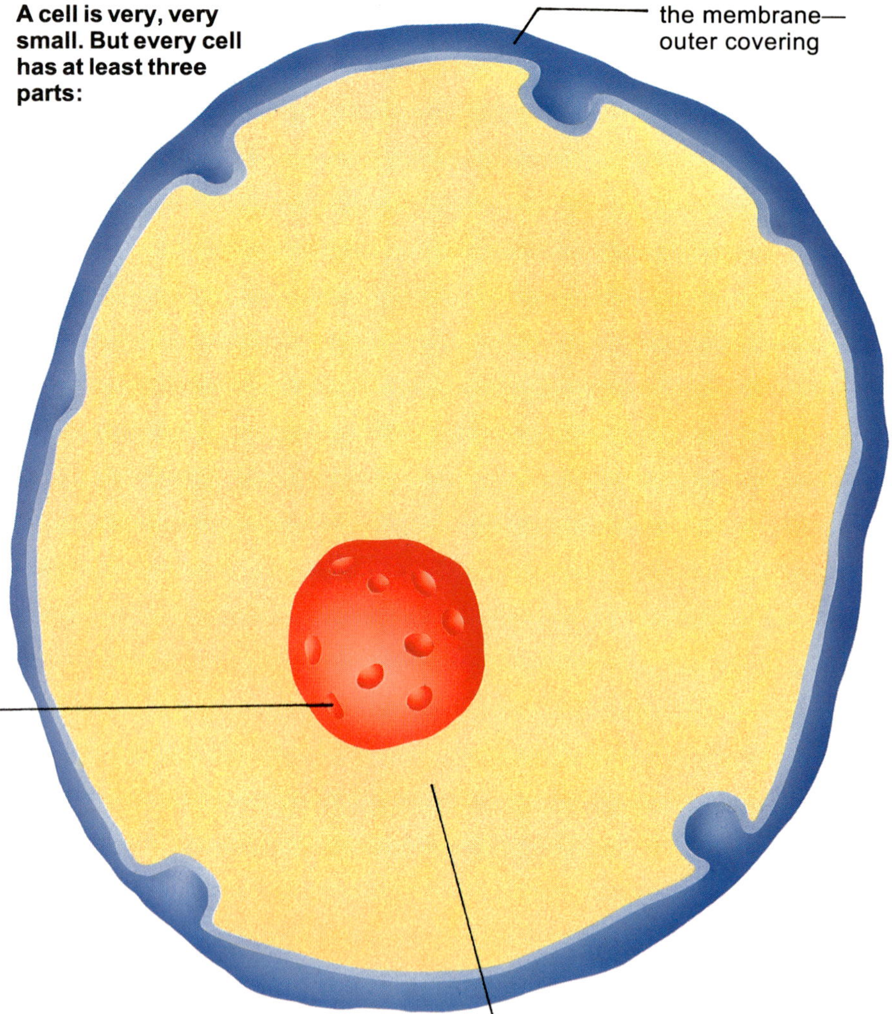

There are different cells in different parts of your body. Here are some of them magnified many times.

bone cells

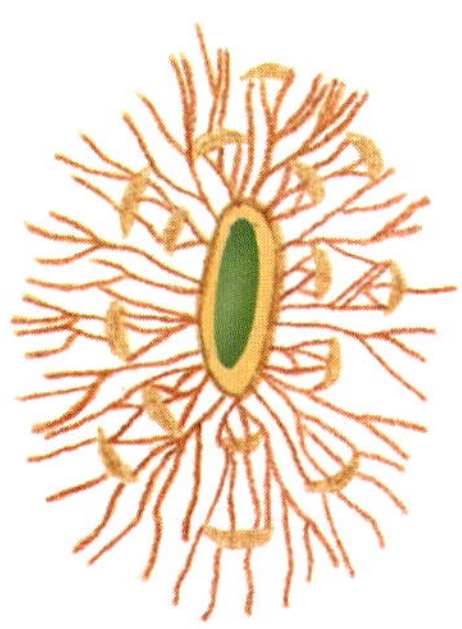

muscle cells

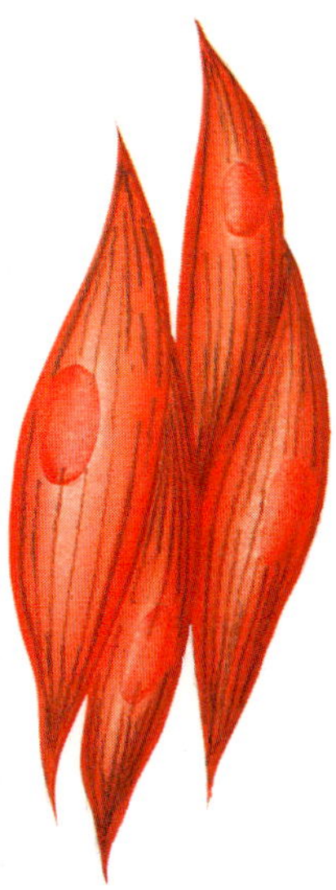

cheek cells

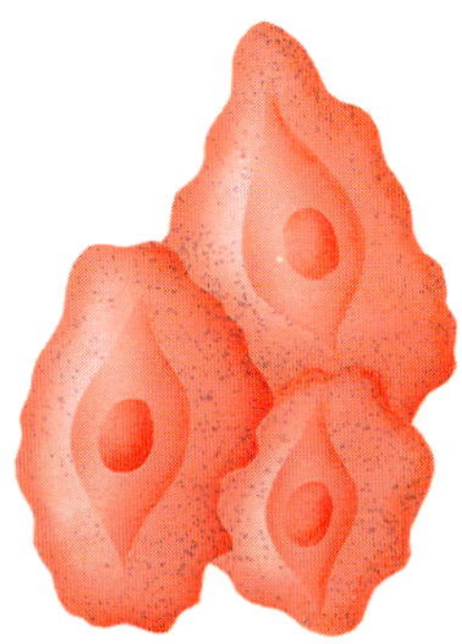

HOW DO CELLS FIT TOGETHER?

Groups of cells make up tissues. For example, muscle cells grouped together make up muscle tissue. Bone cells together make up bone tissue.

The tissues grow in the right way to make organs—working parts with their own special jobs to do, such as the heart and the lungs. An organ may have several different types of tissue in it. For example, the small intestine has tissue which makes juices to help digest food, and muscle to move the food along.

Some cells form what is called connective tissue: it holds the organs in the right place, and joins each organ to the next one.

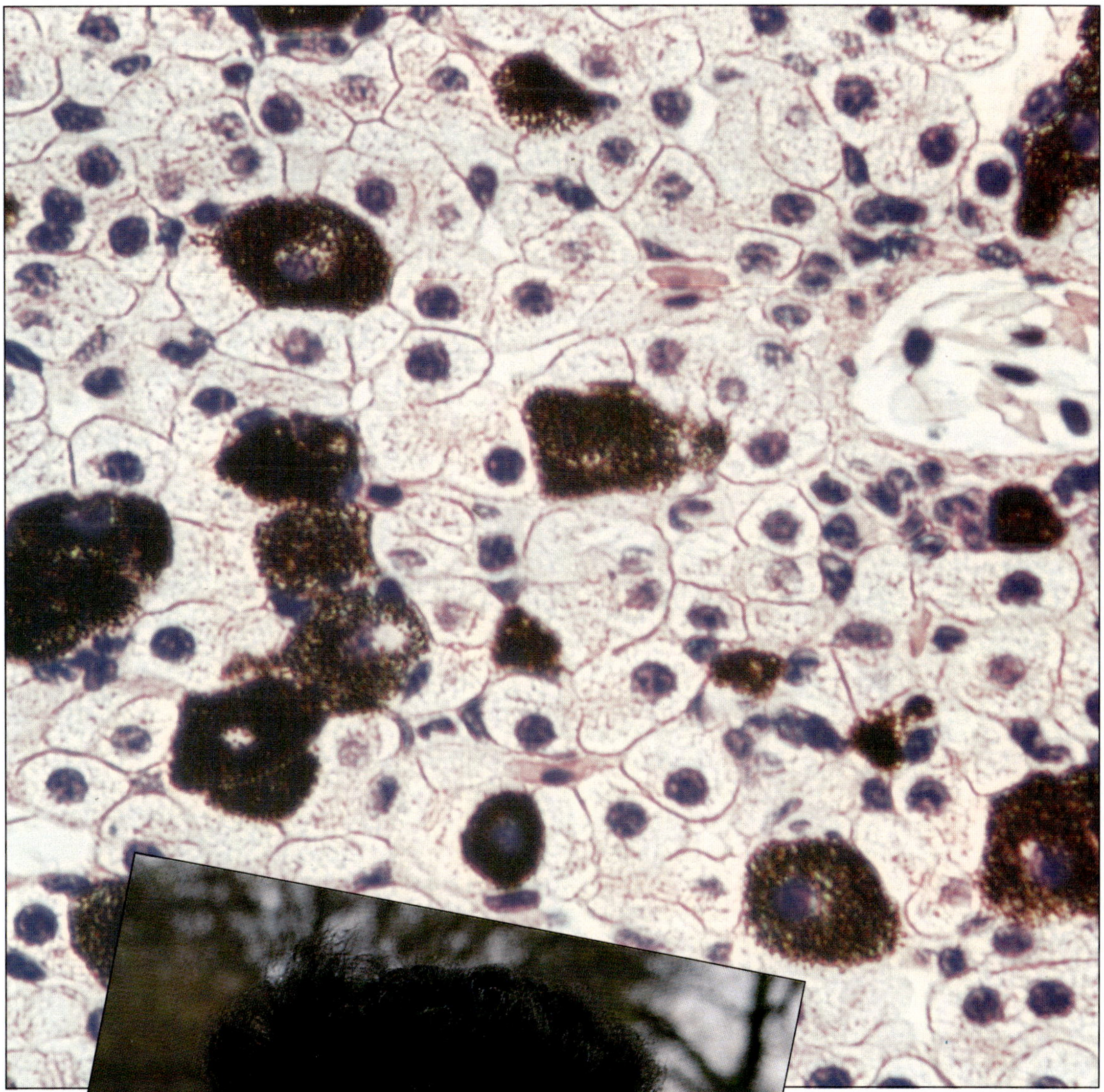

This photograph shows the cells in liver tissue. They are enlarged about 400 times their real size.

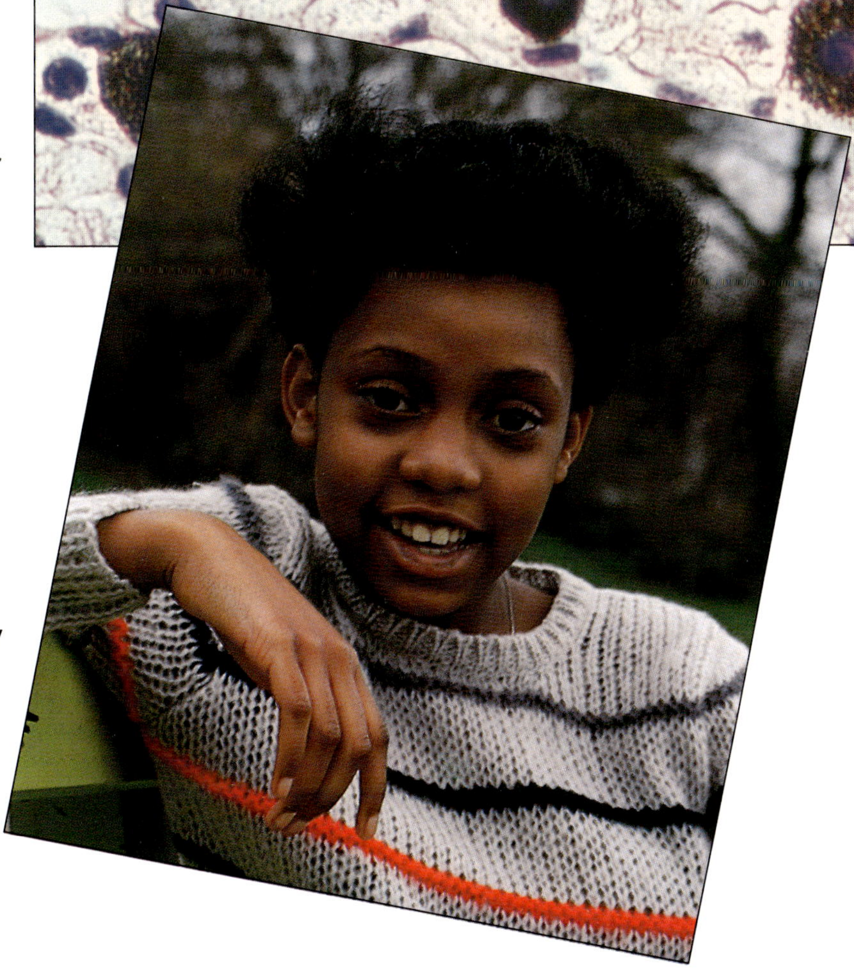

Groups of cells of the same kind make up different types of body tissue. What types of tissue can you see in this picture?

DID YOU KNOW?

Did you know that a person starts life as two cells joining together? A cell from the mother and a cell from the father join together and grow into a human baby.

HOW A BABY IS MADE

Every body begins as a baby, and a baby starts to grow from just two special cells. One cell is from the mother, the other from the father.

Men's bodies are designed so they can become fathers. Women's bodies are designed differently, so they can become mothers. The differences between the bodies are called sex differences, and the ones on the outside are easy to see even in little children.

However, the body parts that are used to make babies only begin to work fully around the time a person becomes a teenager. This time of change is called puberty.

Many people wait a lot longer before taking on the responsibility of having a baby. They still have a lot of growing up of their own to do!

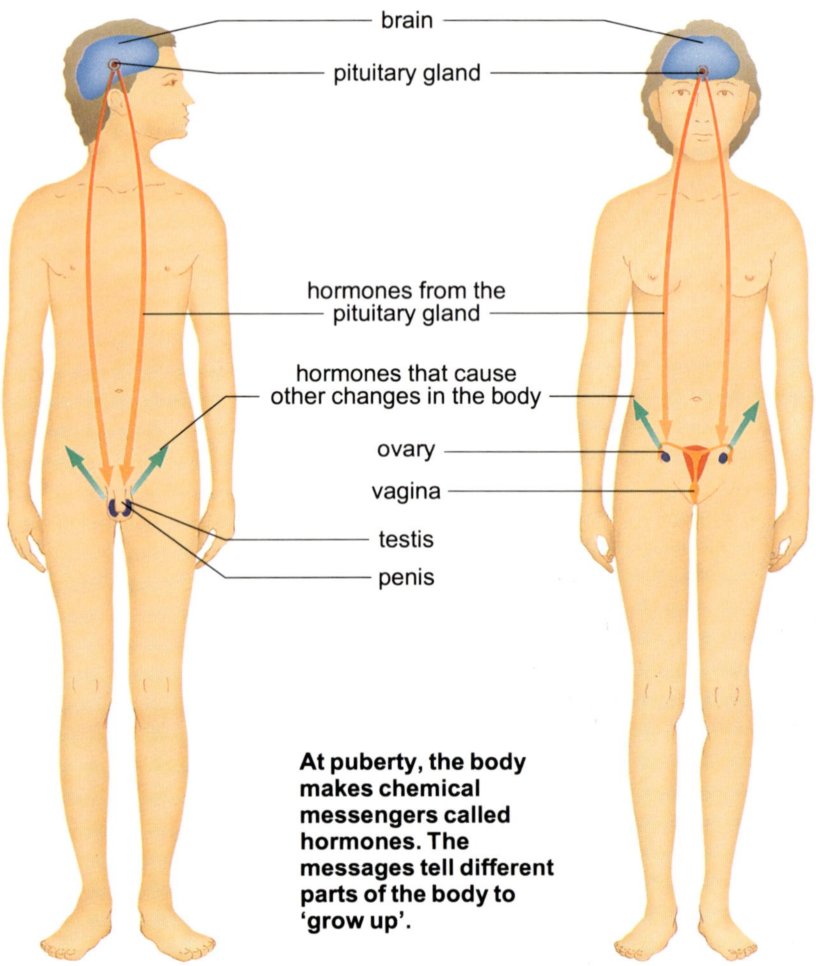

At puberty, the body makes chemical messengers called hormones. The messages tell different parts of the body to 'grow up'.

PUBERTY: GIRLS

Puberty in girls often starts between 11 and 14. Again, chemical messengers get to work. On the outside, girls begin to grow hair between their legs and under their arms. Their breasts begin to grow to a womanly shape. Organs inside the body called ovaries start releasing egg cells—the special cells that the mother provides to make a baby.

The ovaries are linked to another organ, the uterus, which is where a baby can grow. Each month the uterus grows a thicker lining, so it is ready for a baby if it is needed. If it isn't, this thicker lining is shed, along with a little blood.

Girls notice this as bleeding which lasts a few days each month. The bleeding is called menstruation or, more commonly, a period. Girls and women need to wear something that will absorb the blood. One easy solution is pads that have a special sticky strip to hold them inside knickers. Another is to use tiny cylinders of absorbent material called tampons, which slip inside the vagina.

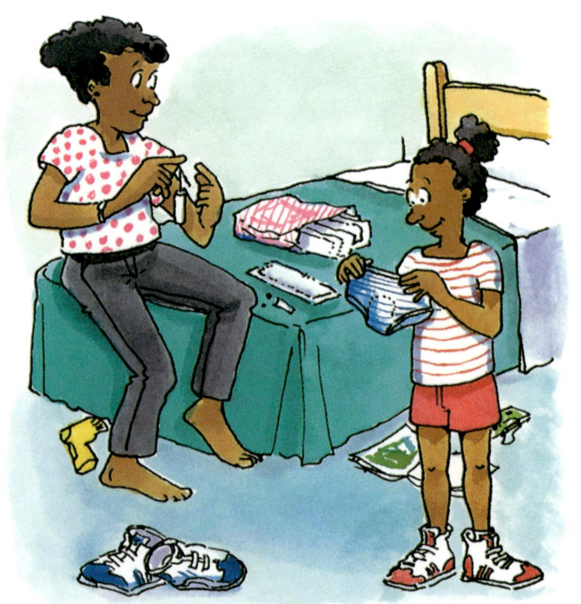

PUBERTY: BOYS

Puberty usually begins in boys when they are between 13 and 16. Chemical messengers in the body, called hormones, cause organs in the scrotum, the testes, to produce sperms. These are the special cells that the father provides to make a baby.

At the same time, other changes begin to take place too. Boys begin to grow hair between their legs, under their arms and on their faces. Their voices 'break' and becomes deep, like a man's.

GETTING TOGETHER

The natural way for an egg and a sperm to meet is when a man and a woman enjoy a specially close and loving relationship. As they cuddle up to each other, the loving feelings they have for each other cause changes in their bodies. The man's penis is made of special tissue that fills up with more blood than at other times and becomes larger and stiff. The woman's vagina gets warm and slippery.

When they are both ready, the man can gently push his penis into the woman's vagina. As they move together while they are close like this, they both enjoy good and loving feelings which get stronger and stronger. When the man reaches a peak of excitement, he fountains a shower of tiny sperms in fluid into the woman's vagina.

The woman can also reach a similar peak of excitement as her body is caressed. The feelings then become less strong, and both partners feel relaxed and happy.

This is sometimes called 'making love'. Another term for it is sexual intercourse. The peak of excitement is called an orgasm.

The sperms swim like tiny tadpoles up through the woman's vagina into her uterus—the place where a baby can grow. As the sperms swim upwards they may meet an egg cell, an ovum. One sperm may join up with the ovum: conception has then taken place. The two joined cells then start to grow into a baby.

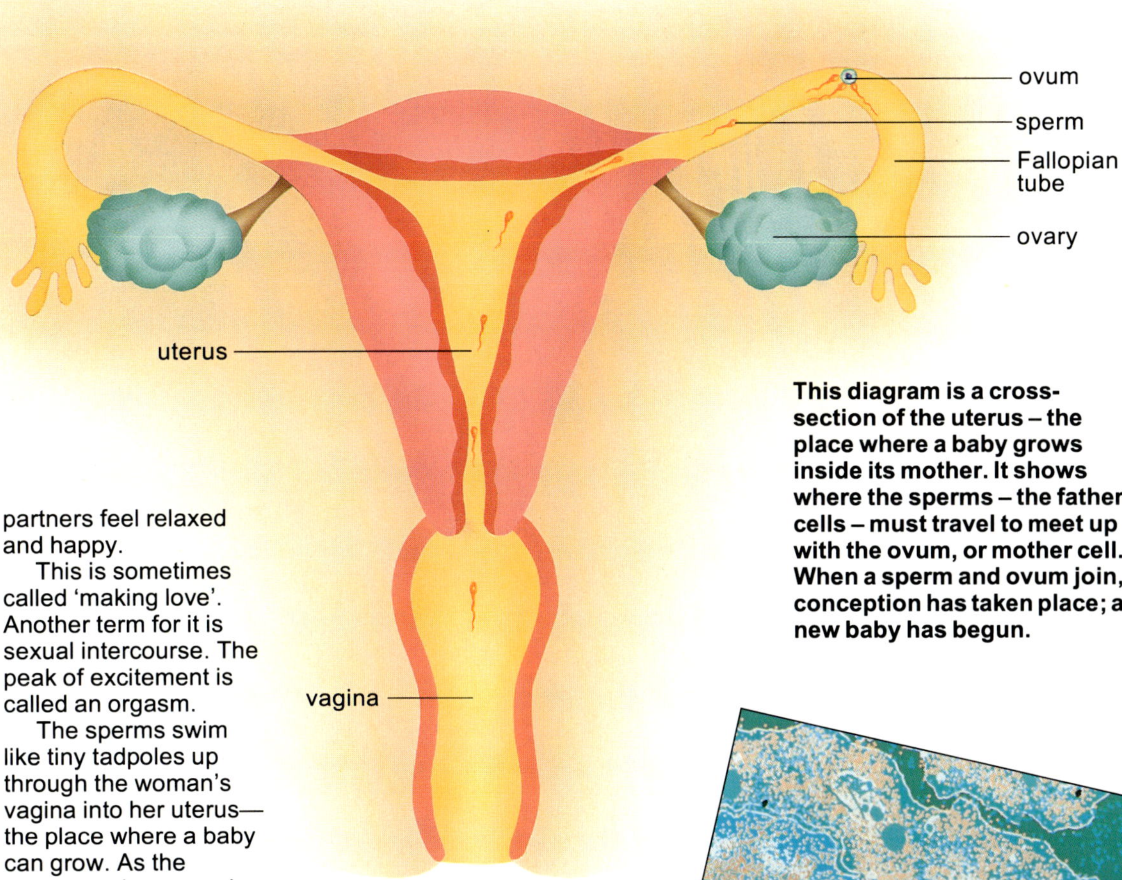

This diagram is a cross-section of the uterus – the place where a baby grows inside its mother. It shows where the sperms – the father cells – must travel to meet up with the ovum, or mother cell. When a sperm and ovum join, conception has taken place; a new baby has begun.

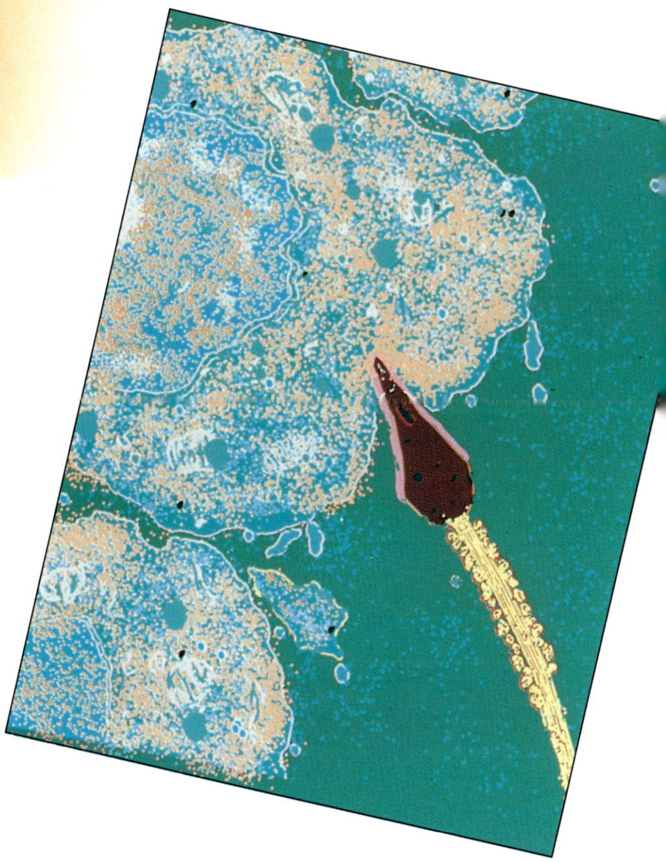

A photograph of a sperm, magnified about 4,000 times, trying to find a way into an ovum. If it succeeds and joins with the mother cell, a new life will begin.

PARTNERS

The special kind of loving that happens between a man and a woman during sexual intercourse makes them feel very close. All over the world, people from many backgrounds feel that this should only happen between people who are married to each other: people who have promised to stay together and take care of each other for all their lives.

The Bible, for example, teaches that God's plan for relationships is for a husband and wife to be completely loyal to each other. That kind of loyalty helps build every part of their friendship, which enables them to love and support each other in everything.

THE BIRTH OF A BABY

When the male sperm cell and the female egg cell meet then something quite amazing happens. Both types of cell have been specially designed so that there are instructions in the nucleus of each that say what sort of person that baby is to grow into.

Sometimes people may say that you look just like someone else in your family. This is because a 'family likeness' is passed down from parents to children in the sperm cell and the ovum cell. So, for example, tall parents are likely to have tall children. You are what you are partly because of what has been passed on to you.

HOW DOES A BABY GROW?

The sperm and ovum join together—this is called 'conception'. Next, the joined cells begin to divide into two and then into four, and so on rapidly until there are lots of cells.

It takes 38 weeks (just over 9 months) for a baby to develop in its mother before it is really ready to be born. During that time the mother is pregnant.

When a sperm joins to an ovum a tiny baby begins to grow in the mother's uterus.

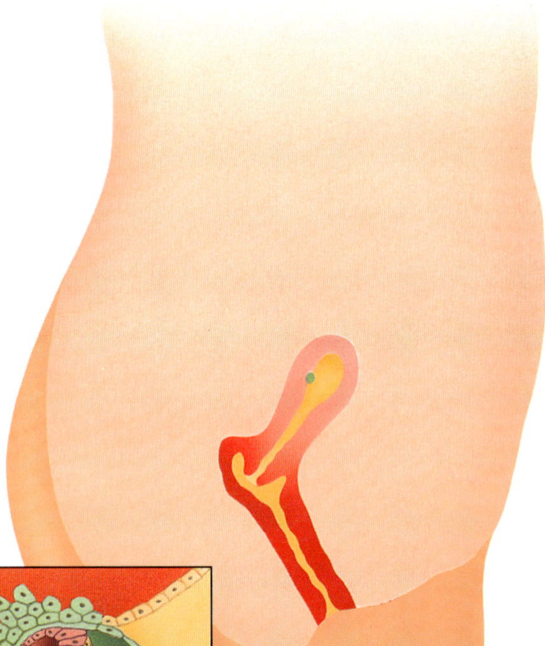

By nine weeks it has tiny arms and legs.

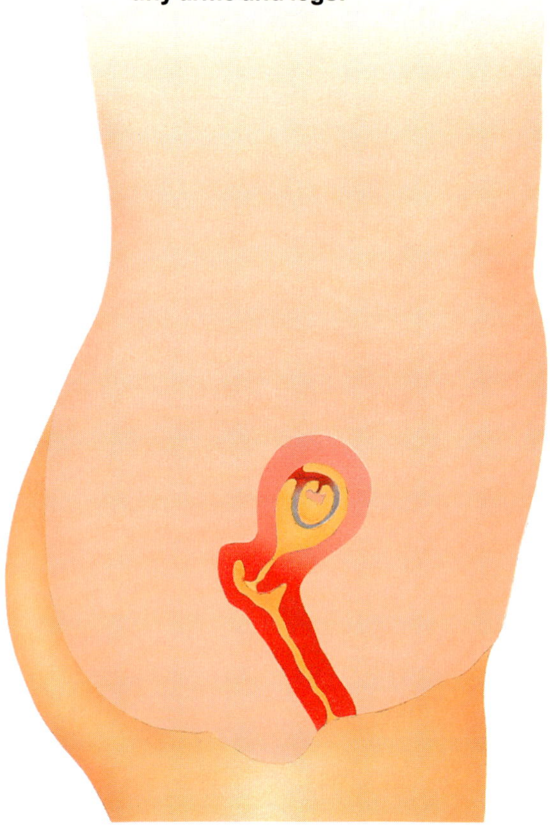

A close-up of the ball of cells that grows from the sperm and ovum. Very soon, some of the cells grow into the wall of the uterus and form the placenta, which controls the supplies of food that the baby gets from its mother. The other cells are the beginning of the new baby.

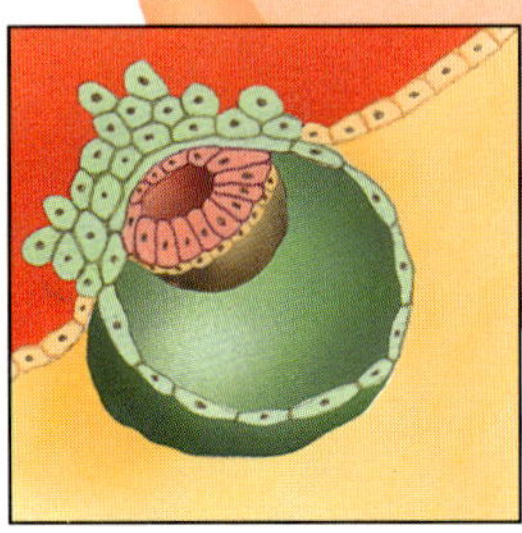

Close-up of a baby-to-be at 9 weeks.

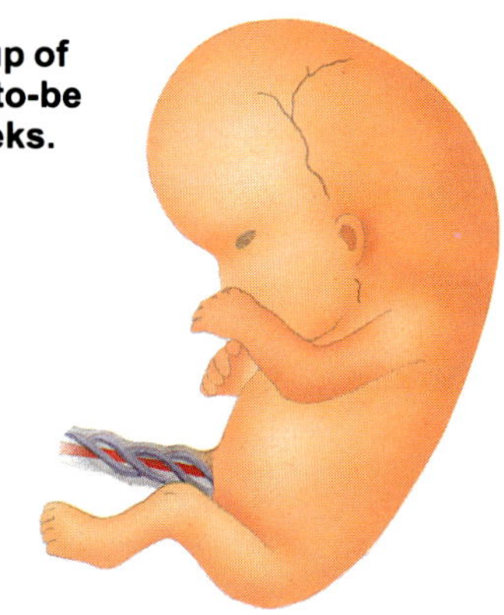

BASIC SUPPLIES

While the baby is in its mother's uterus it is not fed on real food. Instead it gets all it needs from its mother's blood. This supply comes to it through a tube going into its tummy. This tube connects with a special organ called the placenta which grows in the uterus when the baby does.

Once a baby has been born, this connection is no longer needed. The cord is cut by a nurse, or whoever is taking care of the mother while her baby is being born. The stump of the cord soon dries up and falls off, leaving a 'tummy button'.

The placenta slips out of the mother after the birth of the baby. It has done its job.

PLANNING FOR A FAMILY

The act of making love does not always start a baby growing. The woman's egg cell, the ovum, is only at the right stage to join up with a sperm for a few days each month. A couple who want to have a baby need to work out the best time to make love in order to start a baby. Or, if they don't particularly want to have a baby, they may decide to make love at times when conception is less likely.

There are also artificial ways of preventing conception: methods of contraception. For example, there is a device called a condom–a thin rubber sheath that a man can put over his penis when it is stiff, and which catches the sperm and fluid. There are also contraceptive pills.

Some people, such as Roman Catholics and Muslims, forbid the use of artificial contraceptives.

At twenty-four weeks the baby looks like a miniature human being.

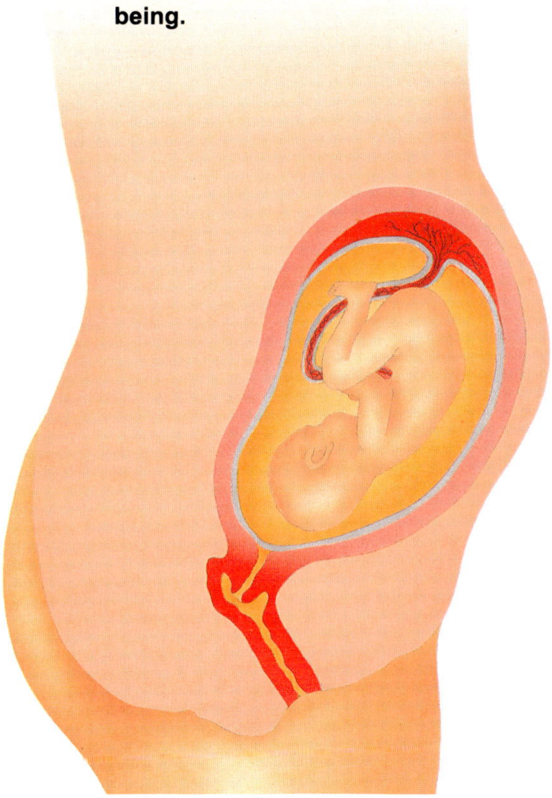

At thirty-six weeks the baby is almost ready to be born.

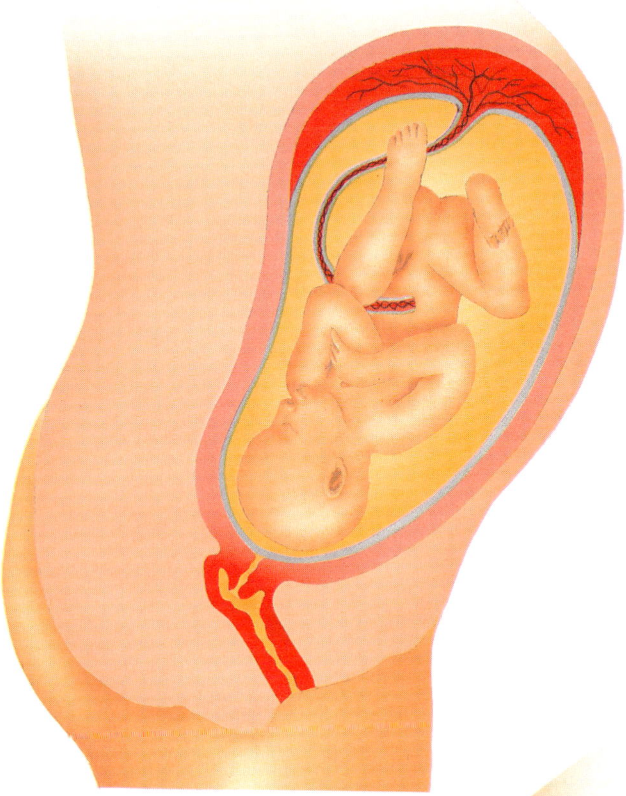

HOW DOES A BABY GET OUT?

When the time comes, the mother knows that her baby is ready to be born. Her uterus is very strong and contains special muscles that are able to push the baby out. When they start to do this she is 'going into labour'. Her vagina stretches to make room for the baby to get out between her legs.

The baby then starts to live by itself outside its mother for the first time. It cries, breathes, and begins to make little sucking movements with its lips. It can drink milk as soon as it is born.

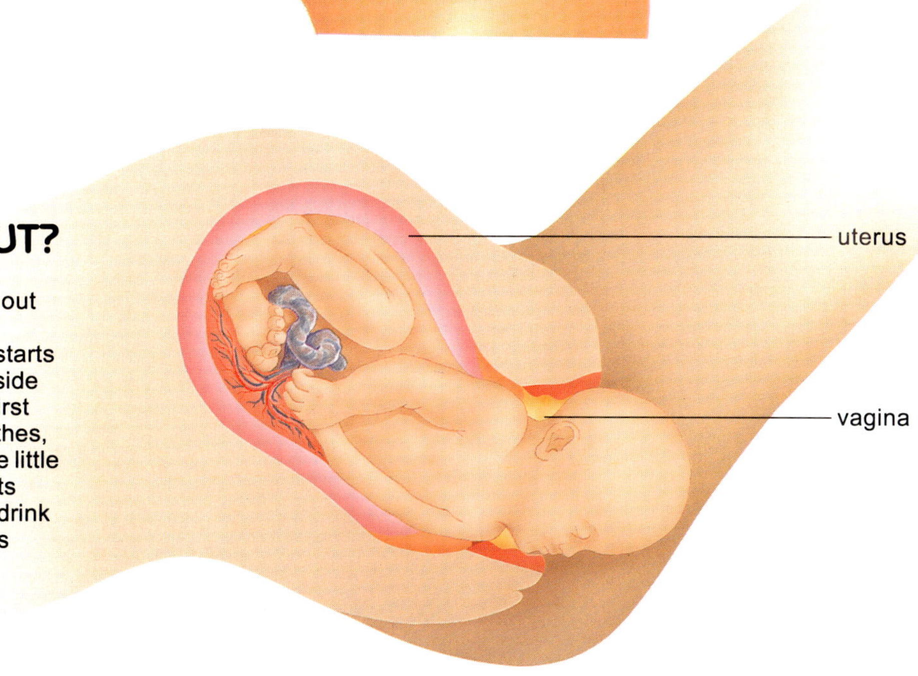

OUTER WRAPPING—THE SKIN

The skin is the largest organ in your body. That's not really a surprise when you think that it covers all round the outside of your body!

Skin is made up of layers of cells to form a tough outer covering. It keeps germs, water and poisons out, keeps moisture and heat in, and stops the body's soft insides from getting hurt.

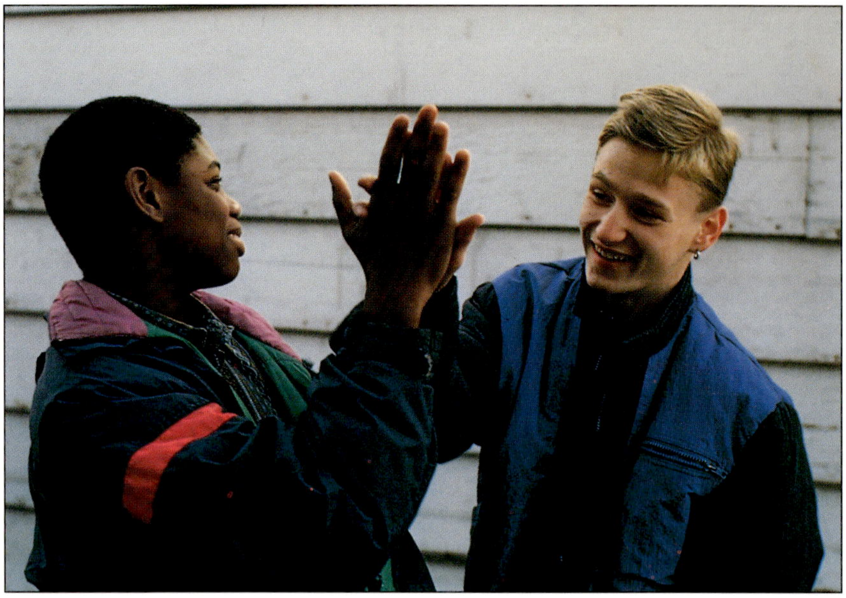

People come in many different skin tones. If you try drawing and colouring people, you will need a wide range of crayons or markers to get the skin colour right. And you'll discover that no one is 'white' or 'black'!

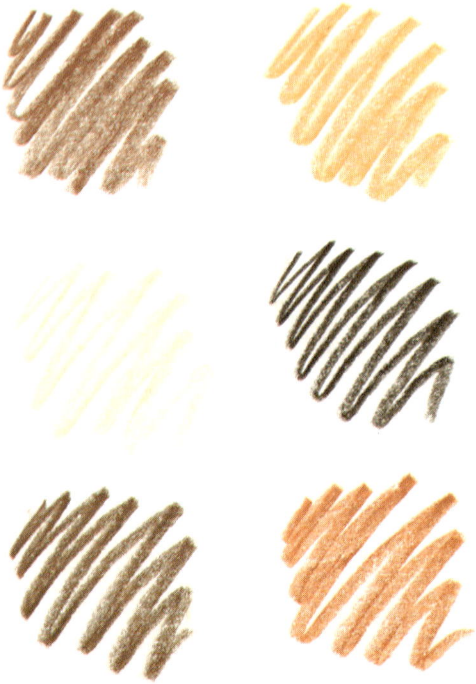

SKINTONES

Everyone's skin contains a brown colouring agent called melanin. This helps to protect the body from the sun's rays.

The different peoples of the world have different amounts of melanin, matched to the amount of sun they would typically get in that part of the world. Those with only a little melanin have light pink skin. Those with a lot have dark brown skin.

Nowadays, people have moved around to different countries, and people with different skin tones live all over the world.

Inside, the organs of the body are the same colour in all people.

SUN SCREEN

Too much sun can harm the skin. It should never be allowed to have so much sun that it burns, and even leaving it exposed so it tans a darker colour can cause damage. People who live in very hot and sunny countries often wear long, loose clothing and a head covering. If you want to leave more of your body bare—as on the beach—then a sunscreen lotion will help protect your skin.

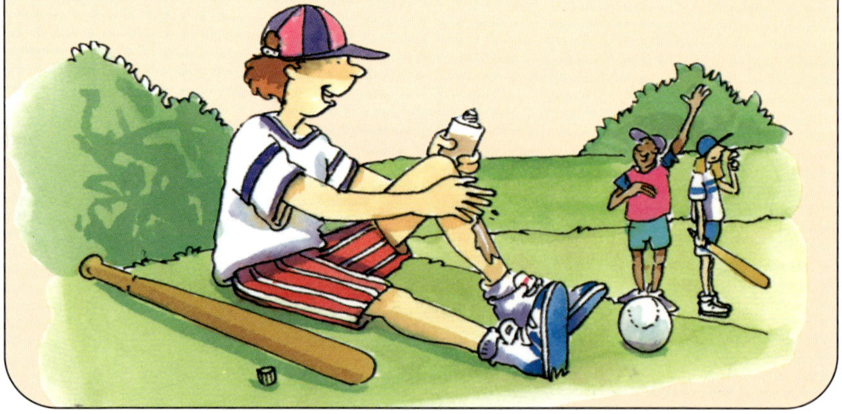

THICK-SKINNED

Did you know that skin is thick in some parts of your body and thin in others? On the soles of your feet the skin is tough and about 6mm thick, to protect the muscles and bones of your feet from pressure. Around your eyes it is very thin—about 0.5mm thick.

CLOSE-UP ON SKIN

Sweat glands in your skin pour out sweat when you are hot. As this liquid (mainly water) evaporates, it takes heat from your body, and so cools you down.

Tiny nerves let you feel things.

Oil glands produce oil to stop your skin drying out.

The outer layer is always being renewed: dead cells flake away and living cells die off and take their place.

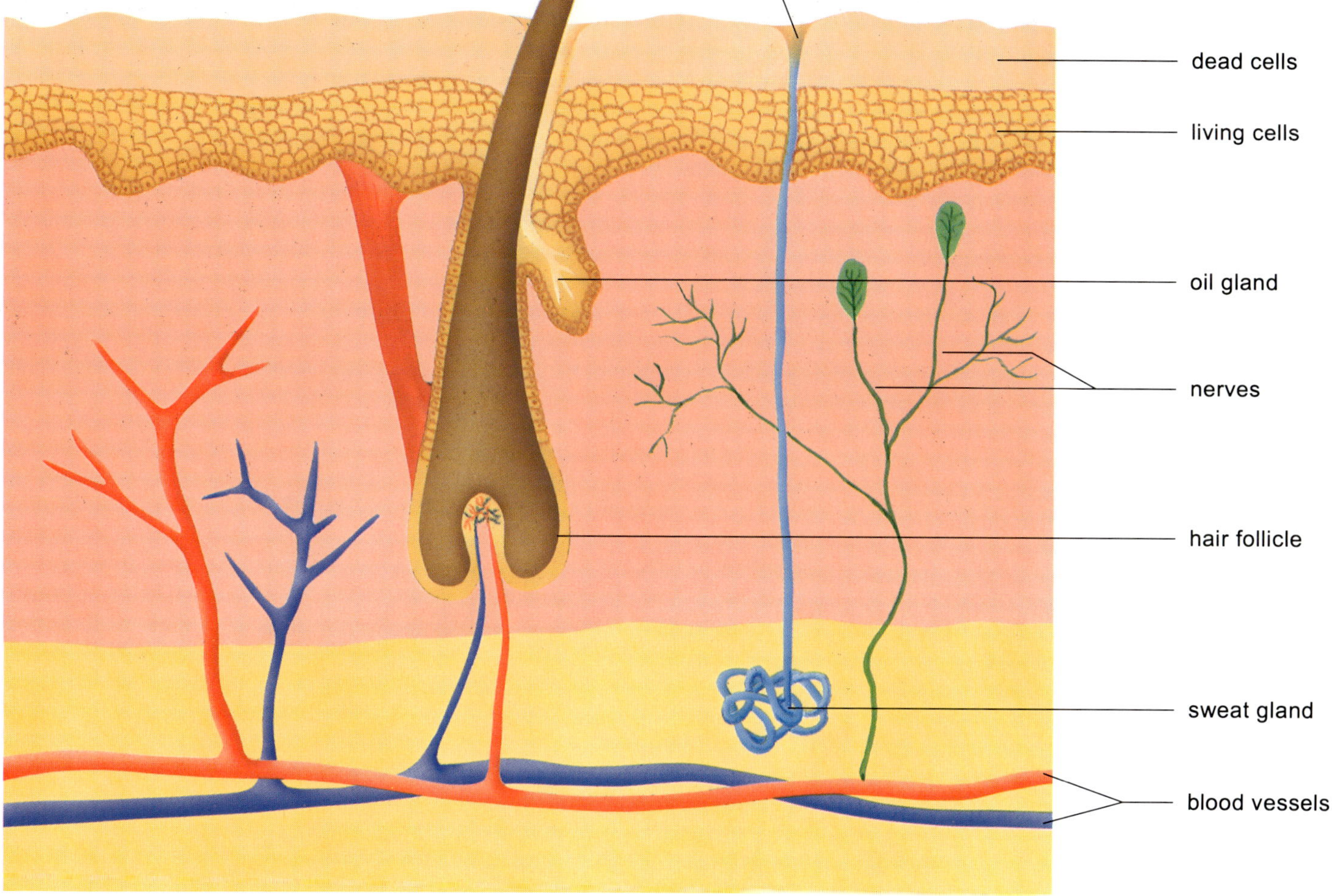

DID YOU KNOW?

Some parts of the skin make a lot of sweat—the armpits and hands, for instance. As the sweat dries, the skin can get smelly. Lots of people put special powder or liquid on their armpits to stop them sweating so much. These products are called anti-perspirants or deodorants.

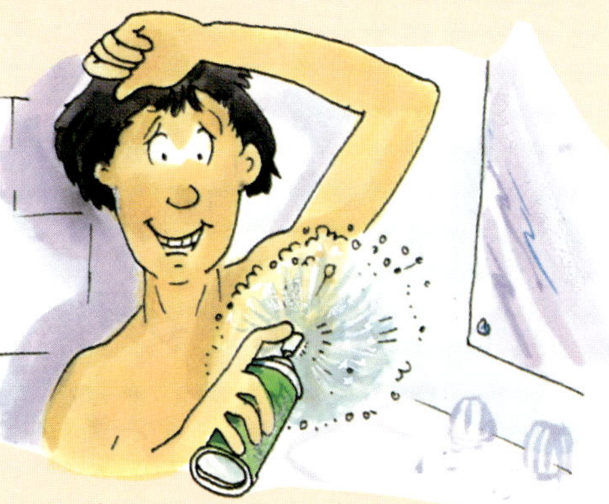

ANCIENT WOUNDS

If you cut yourself your skin is usually very quick to join up again by itself. If the cut is very deep then it may need stitches to hold the cut bits together. This stitching is done by a doctor or nurse.

When the cut is a bad one, the body will make an extra strong join using a slightly different tissue. This is called a scar. It may show a bit, because it is a slightly different colour, but it won't come undone.

KEEP COOL

A burn is really bad news for skin, and needs to be treated carefully—but very urgently. Little burns and scalds (wet burns) are more painful than dangerous. If you get a small burn, try to put the bit that is burned under cool running water for a few minutes. This will take the heat out of the skin, and lessens the damage done.

TIDY TRIMS—HAIR AND NAILS

Hair and nails sometimes seem like extras. People seem to think more about how they look than anything else. But they're very useful, too.

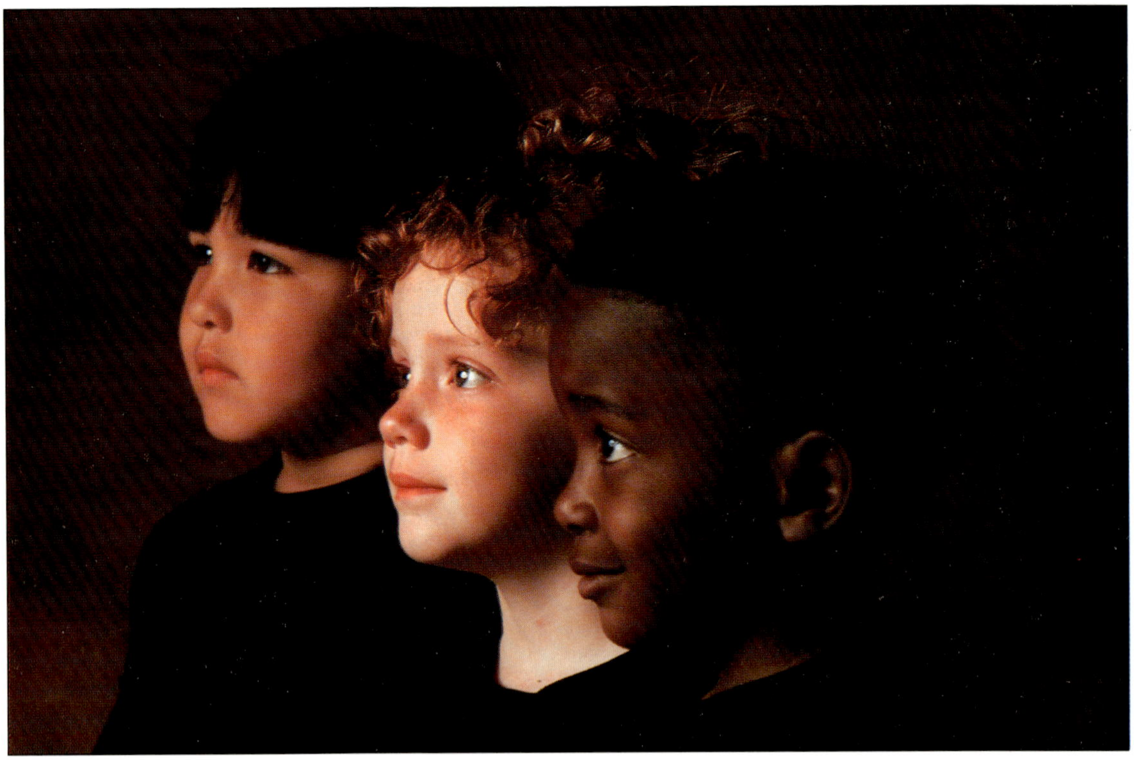

Some people have straight hair, some have wavy hair, and some have curly hair. If you cut through a piece of each type of hair and looked at the cross section under a microscope you would see that each has a special shape. Straight hair is round in cross section; wavy hair is oval, and curly hair is almost rectangular.

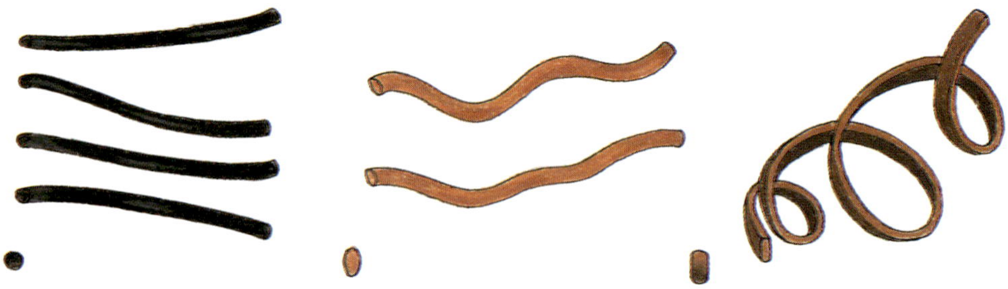

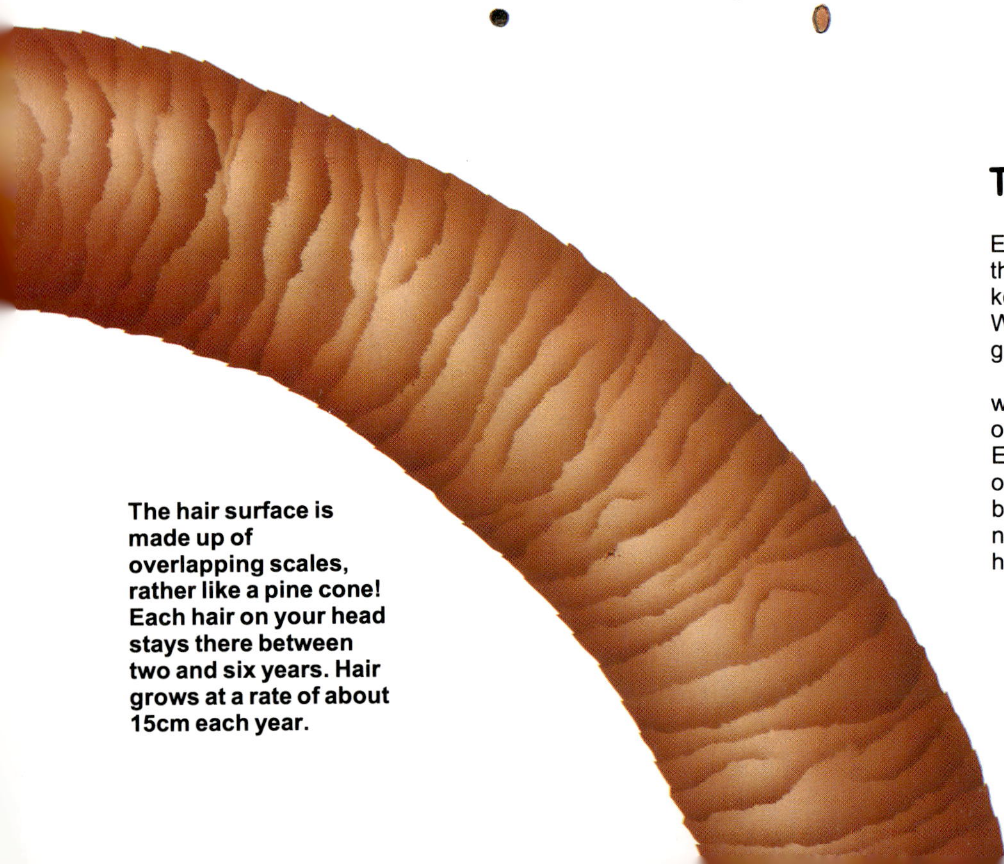

The hair surface is made up of overlapping scales, rather like a pine cone! Each hair on your head stays there between two and six years. Hair grows at a rate of about 15cm each year.

TAKE IT FROM THE TOP

Everyone has hair on their heads. It helps to keep the head warm. Without it, people can get cold very quickly.

Some babies arrive with lots of hair, though others are born bald. Either way, by the end of their first year, most babies will have some noticeable hair on their heads.

A person's hair may change while they are growing up. For example, fair hair may grow darker. Fine hair may thicken up, and perhaps develop some curl.

By the time a person is in their teens, these early changes will all be over.

CLASSY CLAWS

Nails grow best if they are trimmed with scissors. If they are bitten really short for a long time—like years—they may not grow back to the shape they were before.

ON THE NAIL

Nails, on the ends of your toes and fingers, stop these ends from getting grazed or hurt.

Nails are made of special skin, which is hard and tough. They grow up under the surrounding skin from just about your last toe or finger joint. Nails grow at the rate of around 6mm every month. If you have been ill, then you may see little white patches on your nails.

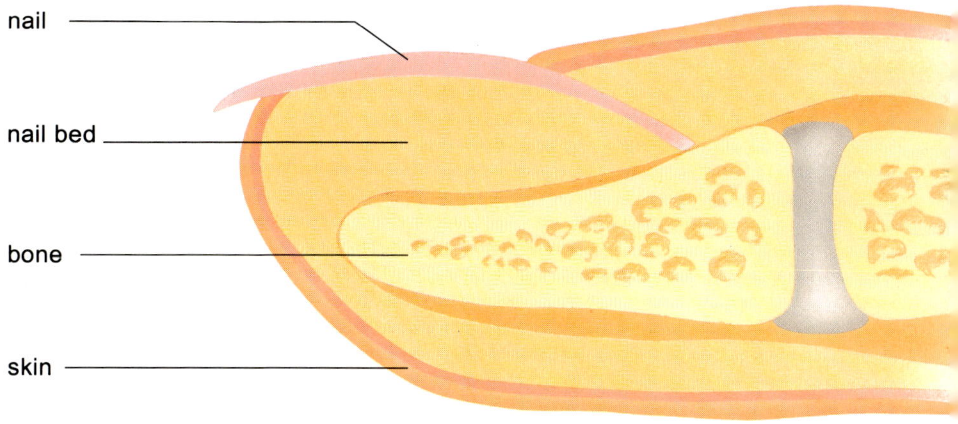

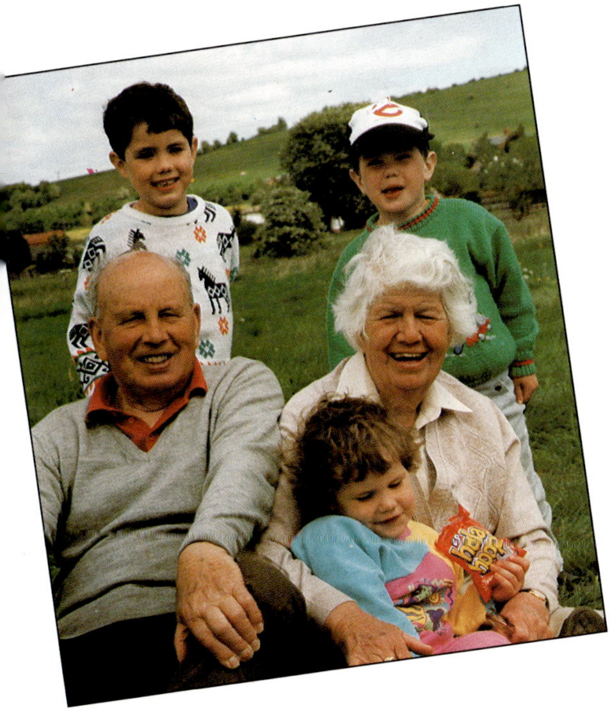

SAFETY FIRST

However you like to wear your hair, do remember to put safety first. That means keeping your hair out of your eyes when you need to see clearly—riding your bicycle, for example. It also means keeping it back when it might otherwise swing forward and get tangled up with what you're doing. So keep it back, or under your hat, when preparing food or working with any sort of machinery, or when you're near an open flame.

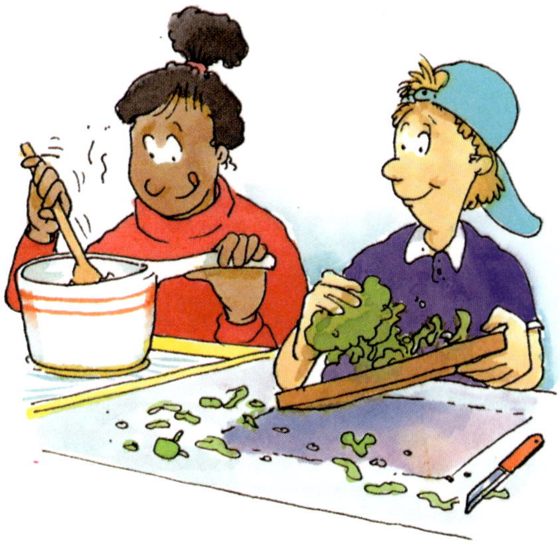

KEEP YOUR HAIR ON!

Other changes take place as a person grows older. Some men go bald. This can happen any time, from the early twenties onwards. Both men and women find that their hair turns grey or white as they grow older. This process can also begin in the twenties and thirties, but more often when a person is older than that.

The tendency to go bald or to go grey is passed down from parent to child. So it is possible to work out what is likely to happen to your hair as you grow older by looking at your parents.

HAIR DOS

- Keep your hair and scalp clean—and you'll help keep them healthy. Washing once a week with a mild shampoo is usually enough. Greasy hair needs more!
- Keep it trimmed. Hair isn't 'alive', and as it grows older, it can begin to split from the ends upwards. Trimming it will help stop this happening. Even if you are growing your hair, you'll need a trim from time to time to keep your hair in good condition.
- If your scalp seems very itchy, ask to see a doctor, to find out what the problem is. It may be something to do with the skin on your head, or perhaps little creatures called lice have taken up residence. They are always quick to hop on any head that they get near, and they do like a nice clean home. Whatever the cause of itchiness, a special shampoo is likely to clear it up.

TEETH

If only you didn't have teeth, there wouldn't be all that tooth-cleaning to do...

But teeth are very useful: designed to let you bite off bits of food and chew into soft pieces you can swallow.

When babies are born, they don't need teeth because they suck milk. But after a few months a baby starts to 'teethe' and baby teeth or 'milk' teeth grow in. These milk teeth are small enough to fit a child's small mouth. But as a person grows, adult teeth grow and push the milk teeth out.

Adults have 28 teeth. Four more teeth usually come in at the back when people are in their late teens. They are called wisdom teeth—because they come at an age when a person is meant to be grown up and wise. But they don't always come through. And they're not a sign of wisdom!

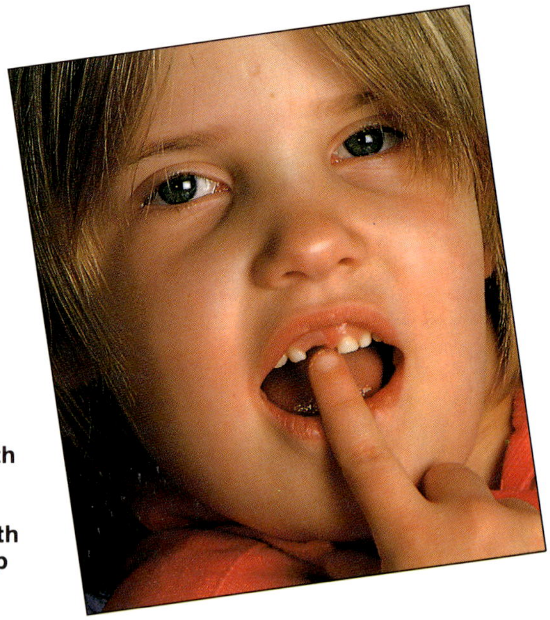

As you get older, your first teeth need to be replaced with the teeth you will have as an adult. As these grow, they gradually push your first teeth out, sometimes leaving a gap for a while.

Teeth are designed for special jobs.

The front teeth, called incisors, are perfect teeth for cutting.

The canine teeth are excellent for gripping and tearing.

At the side are pre-molars, and molars are at the back. They are designed for grinding food.

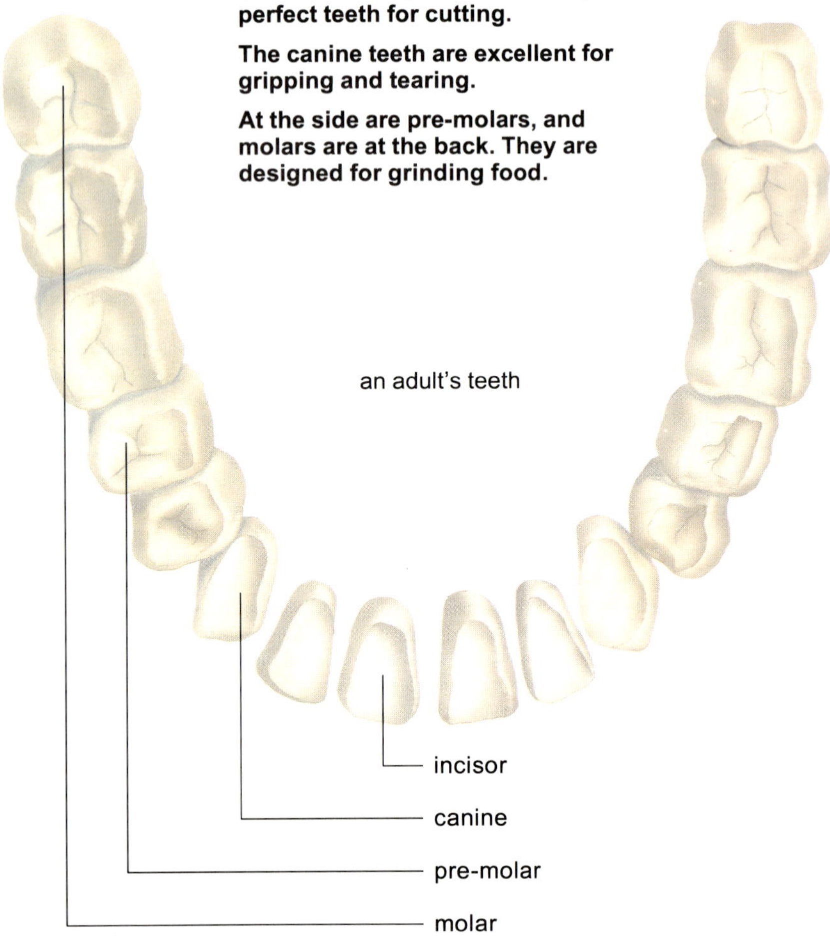

an adult's teeth

LINE UP!

Sometimes teeth do not grow in an even line. Some unevenness is fine: it gives you a distinctive smile. Other times it leaves your teeth in awkward positions that mean you can't bite as well, or can't keep your teeth clean easily. Dentists may advise that you wear a device called a brace. It has to be worn for a long time—months, or years—to get the teeth to grow in the best position for your mouth.

It can be a nuisance to deal with a brace, but when it's over you'll have prize-winning pearlies in your mouth. So even while you wear it, keep practising the smile!

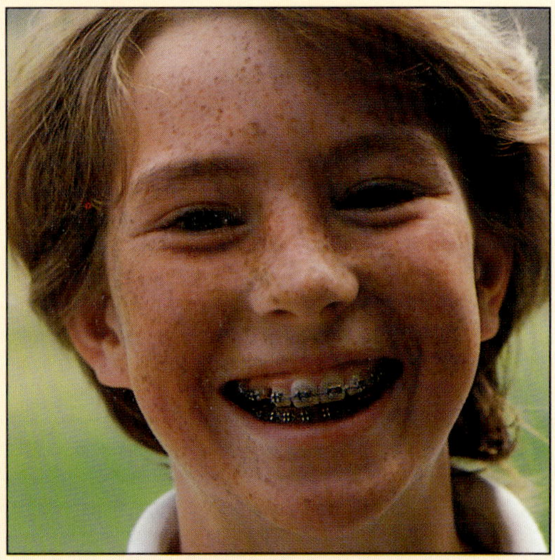

WHAT A PAIN

It is important to look after your teeth. And although brushing your teeth can be dull, it is vital to take the time to clean off the sugars that get left on them. Otherwise, germs begin to flourish in the sugar, and make the tooth covering—enamel—go bad and decay. That looks ugly, and if left untreated it can make the teeth very painful.

It's also important to avoid snacking on sweet and sugary foods, which simply puts sugar back on the teeth.

Regular visits to the dentist are a good idea. That way any problems can be spotted early and put right more easily.

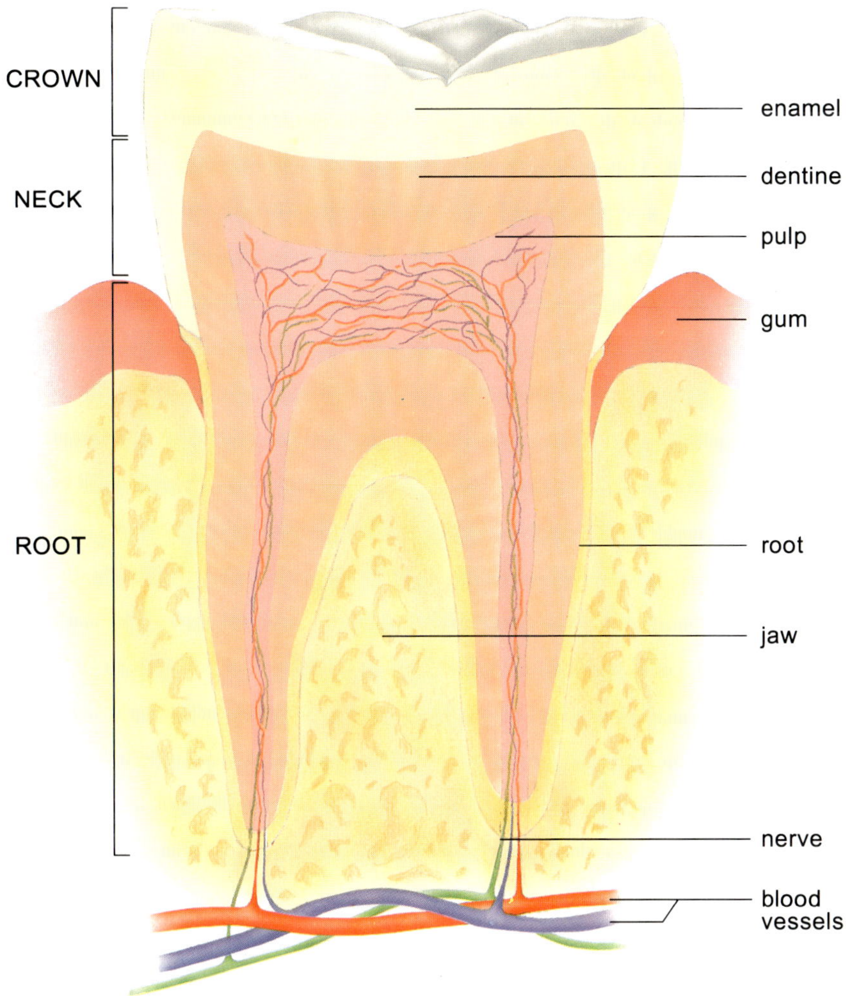

All teeth are covered by an outer protective coat of enamel. Under this is dentine, which is hard and makes up most of the tooth. In the centre is the pulp containing nerves and blood vessels. The tooth aches when something is wrong in the centre, and the nerve sends a message to the brain which makes you feel pain.

Nearly two-thirds of each tooth is embedded in the jaw, which is part of the skull.

Gums are very important in protecting the roots of the teeth from decay. A good clean will look after them too.

THE ULTIMATE TOOTH-CLEANING JOB

Here's how to do a perfect job of cleaning your teeth. The whole thing will take about five minutes. Get into the habit of doing a perfect job every night.

- Take a piece of dental floss. Hold one end in each hand, and use the bit in the middle to clean between your teeth, with a gentle sawing motion. Wipe the floss clean on tissue as you go.
- Chew a plaque-disclosing tablet, which marks bright red the areas that need to be brushed clean. Then put a pea-sized blob of fluoride toothpaste on your toothbrush. Brush, brush, brush, with a movement up and down, to get the teeth and gums clean. Expect to take three minutes at this.
- Rinse your mouth clean with water. If you wish, rinse out again with a fluoride mouthwash.

A quicker brush after every meal will help keep your teeth free from the sugars that let decay get going.

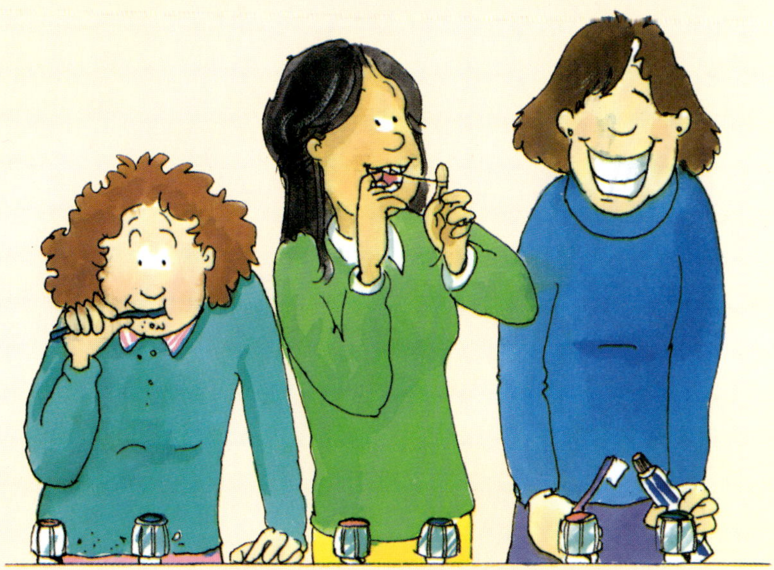

INSIDE INFORMATION—THE BRAIN

People often say that someone is 'brainy' because they are good at school work. But all people are brainy, because they all have a brain!

Without a brain you wouldn't be able to do anything. Your brain makes you able to think; it helps you to learn, and to remember; and it makes sure that all the different parts of you work together.

WHAT DOES THE BRAIN LOOK LIKE?

The human brain looks like a big walnut. It has two halves, which are joined together, and it is grey and craggy.

If you simply took a look at the human brain, you'd never believe all the wonderful things it does—it doesn't look very impressive. But your brain is better than the best computer ever invented. It is more intricate, works faster and is cleverer. No computer has as many functions as the human brain.

WHERE IS THE BRAIN?

Your brain is inside your head, where it is protected by your skull—the bone that gives your head its shape.

WHAT DOES THE BRAIN DO?

Every year scientists find out more about how the human brain works, but they still don't know everything about it.

Information is fed to the brain by nerves from all the different parts of your body. Then instructions are sent to the body down other nerves.

Special parts of your brain receive the information that is fed to it by your five senses: sight, hearing, touch, taste and smell. Your brain can store this information away, so that you remember what was recorded in the brain and can use it in the future.

Your brain does lots of other important things too. It controls what is happening inside you. For example, it controls your body's heating system, making sure it stays at a good level, and it also controls the amount of fluid in your blood so that you have exactly the quantity that is best for you.

Different parts of the brain have different jobs to do.

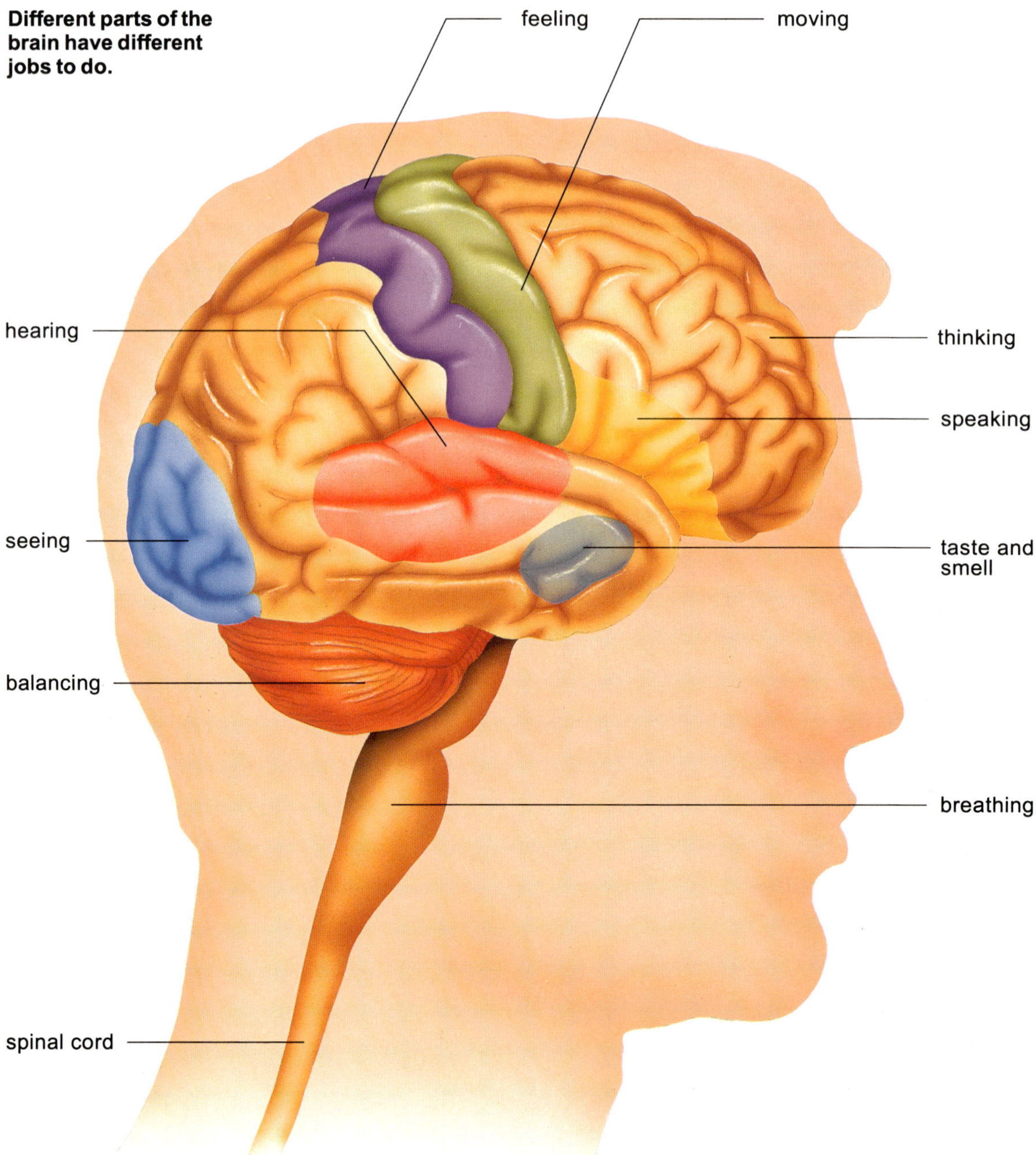

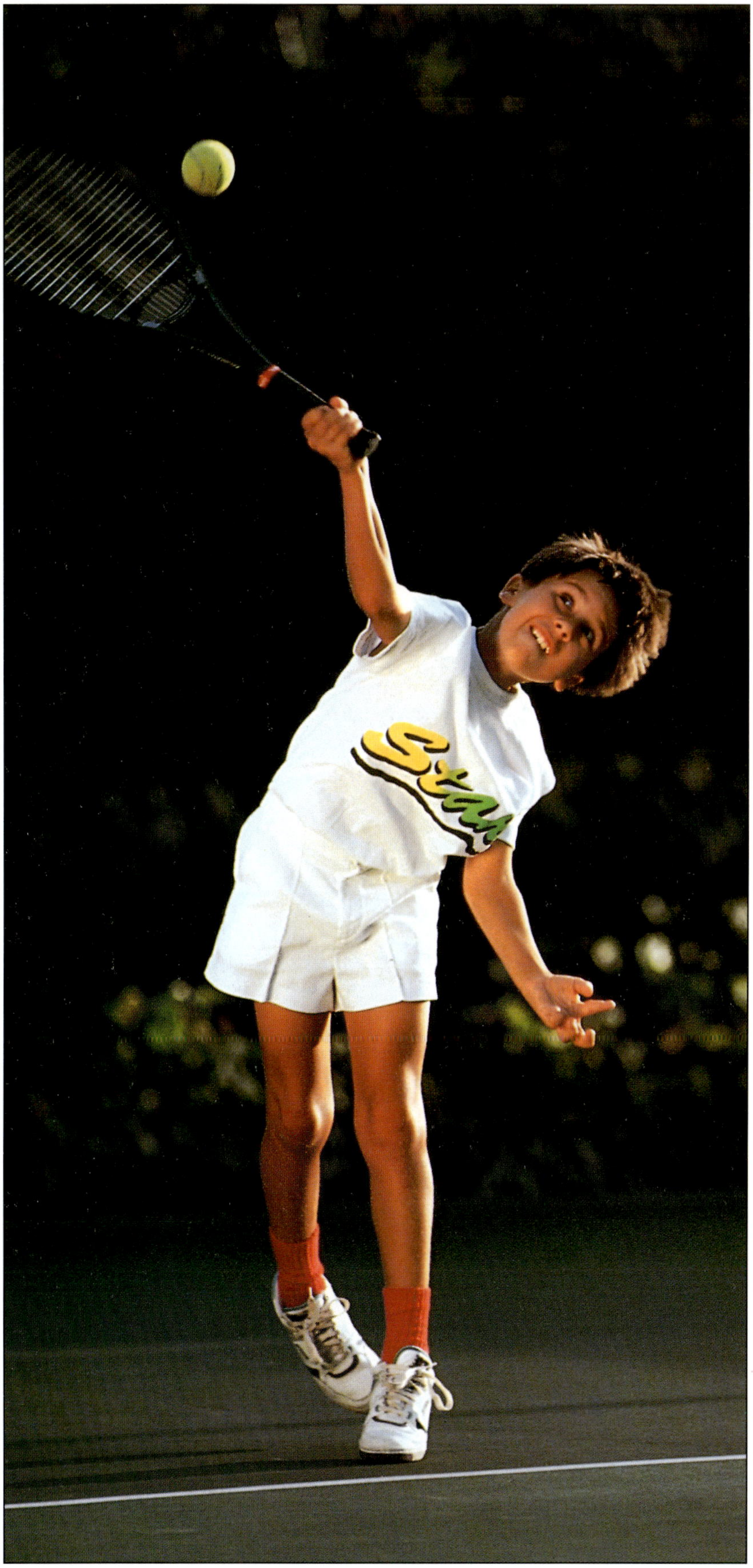

TEAM UP WITH YOUR BRAIN!

Exciting things happen in your brain. You may decide, 'I want to be good at gym!' You think that in your brain. Then your will—the something inside you which decides that you *will* do something because you really want to—encourages you to start practising.

Your brain then helps you remember how to balance, and then makes each muscle work with the others so that you move easily. Your brain helps you to train your muscles and to learn by practising how to control your body and make it do what you want it to do.

Every kind of activity people do requires brain power – physical activities just as much as 'thinking' activities.

SLEEP TIGHT

When you sleep your body and brain rest. Your breathing slows down and your brain works in a different way from its awake state. But while most of your muscles relax during sleep, some work hard. For instance, your eyelid muscles work to keep your eyes closed.

Dreams happen to everyone, every night, but most dreams aren't remembered. If you are woken during a dream you will usually remember it. Nobody knows why we dream, but some people think it helps to sort out in our minds things that happen while we are awake.

MESSAGES TO HEADQUARTERS—NERVES

All over your body is a network of nerves, carrying messages backwards and forwards all the time. It works incredibly fast. As a result, your brain knows almost instantly what's happening to all parts of you—even your littlest toe far away!

The system is also needed for all the everyday things you do: walking, eating, playing, and staying away from things that hurt.

A long bundle of nerve tissue runs from the brain down the back. This is called the spinal cord. It is quite soft, but is housed in a channel in the spine, so it is well protected.

It's helpful to think of the spinal cord as a tree trunk, with nerves branching off from it and going to other parts of the body. These nerves divide again and again, like twigs, so there are tiny nerves reaching into every part of your body. It's also a message center, where messages are received and sent out automatically.

The central nervous system. Nerves go to every part of the human body.

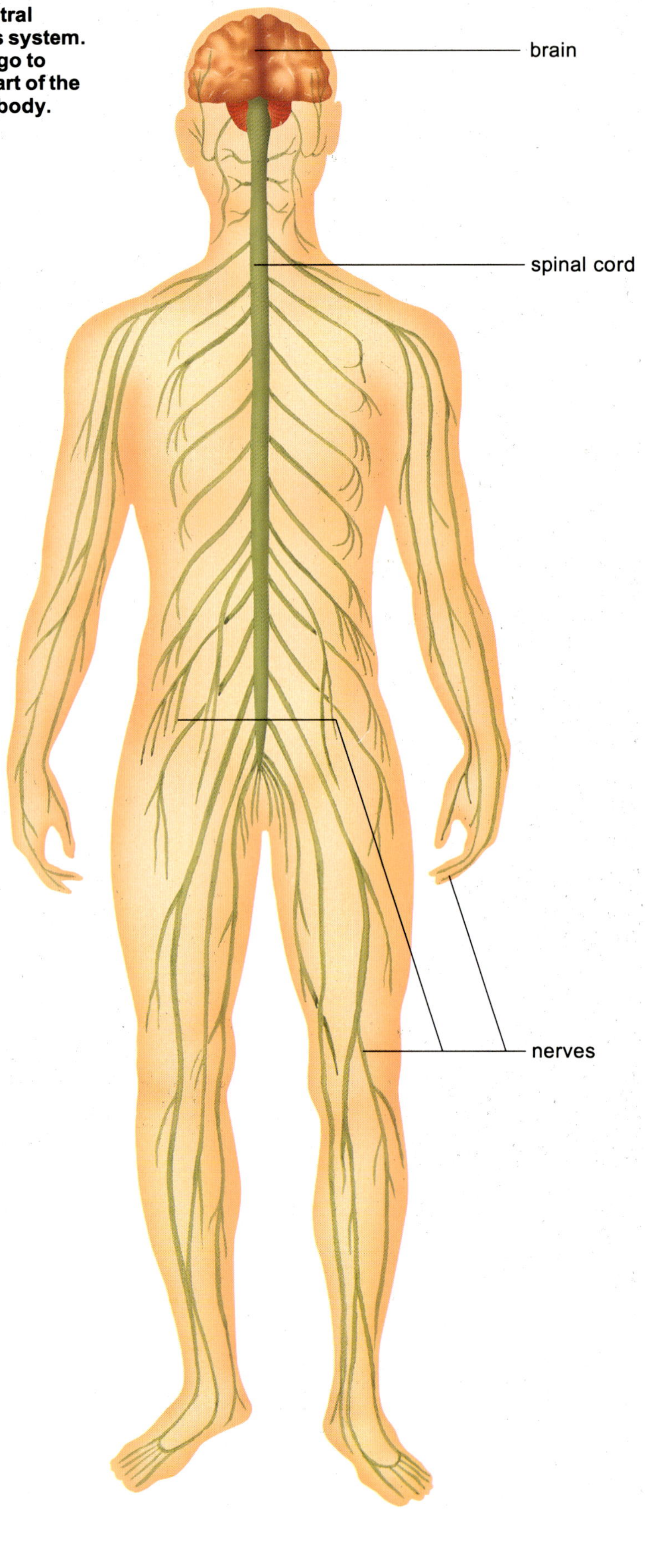

HOLD STEADY!

When your body feels pain, the automatic response is to move away from it. For example, you would normally let go of a pin if you happened to prick yourself on it. But you can steel yourself to sit still when you know a doctor needs to give you an injection.

Sometimes, however, you cannot stop the automatic reaction. For example, if something gets into your windpipe, you cannot stop coughing. Your body knows it is vital to shift it.

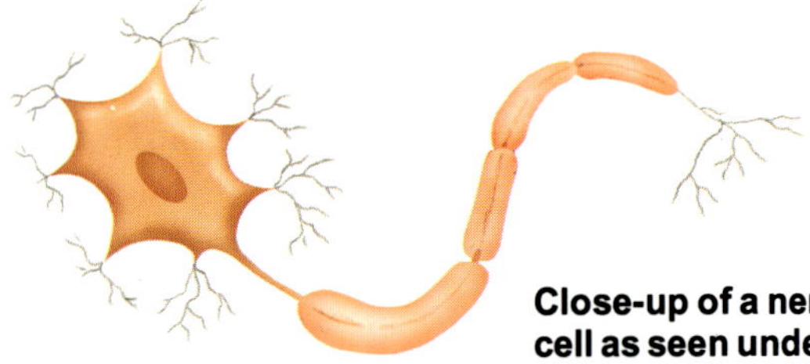

Close-up of a nerve cell as seen under a microscope.

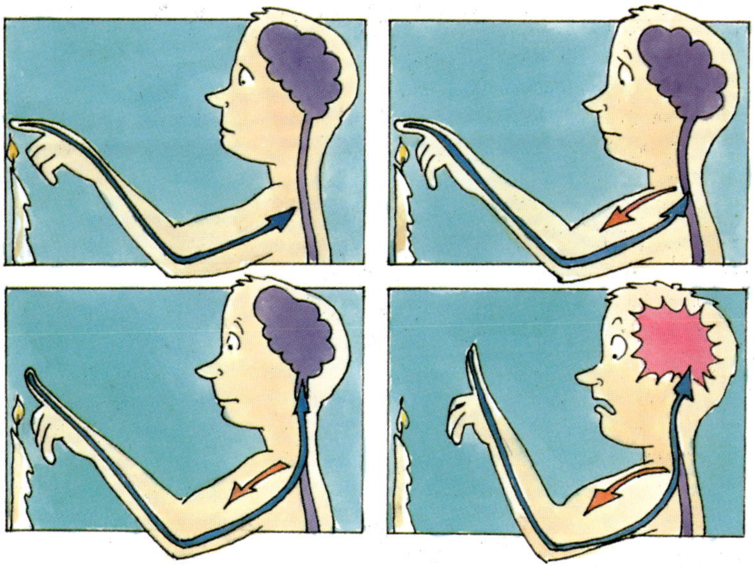

In this situation nerves in your finger send a rapid message. An automatic message is sent back from the spinal cord, which tells you to move your finger *before* the message gets to the brain!

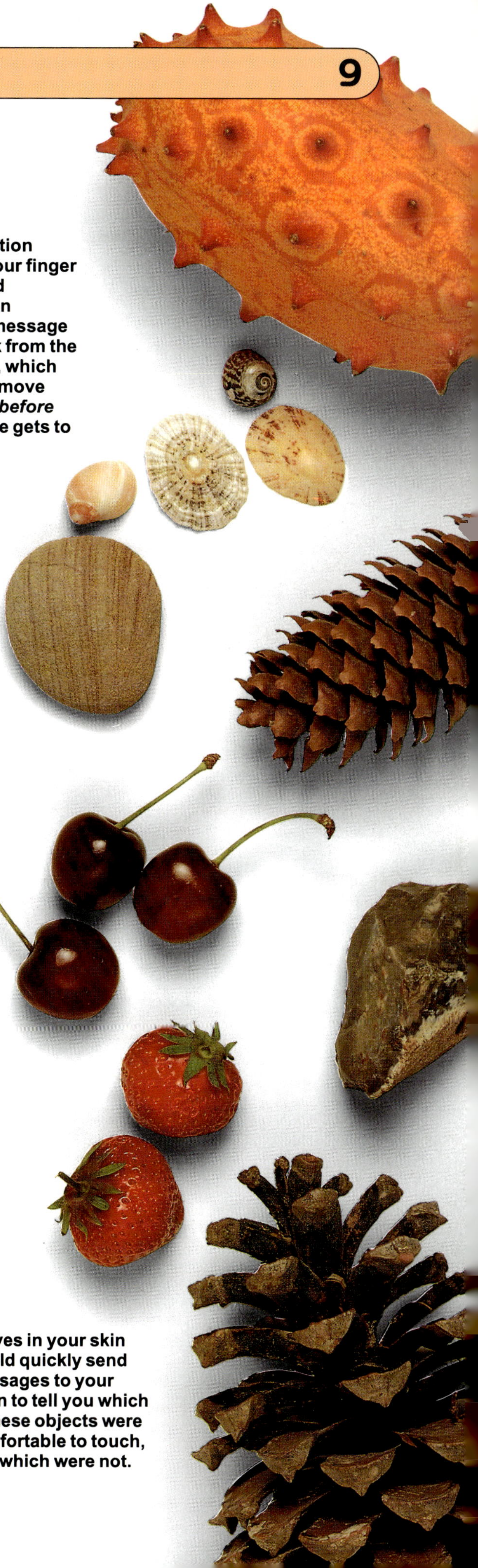

DON'T STICK YOUR NECK OUT!

The spinal cord passes through the backbone and up through the neck to the brain. It is so important that injuries to it can be very serious indeed.

Injuries to the spinal cord happen most often at the neck. For example, if people dive into shallow water they may hit their heads on the bottom of the pool, lake or sea, and break their necks. In a car crash, the people in the cars may have their heads jerked back by the sudden change in speed. In either case, the bones in their necks may be broken apart.

Sometimes this only bruises the cord. Other times it might break it altogether. This means that the messages that usually tell the body what to do cannot get through. As a result, the brain cannot get the body to move. This is called being paralyzed.

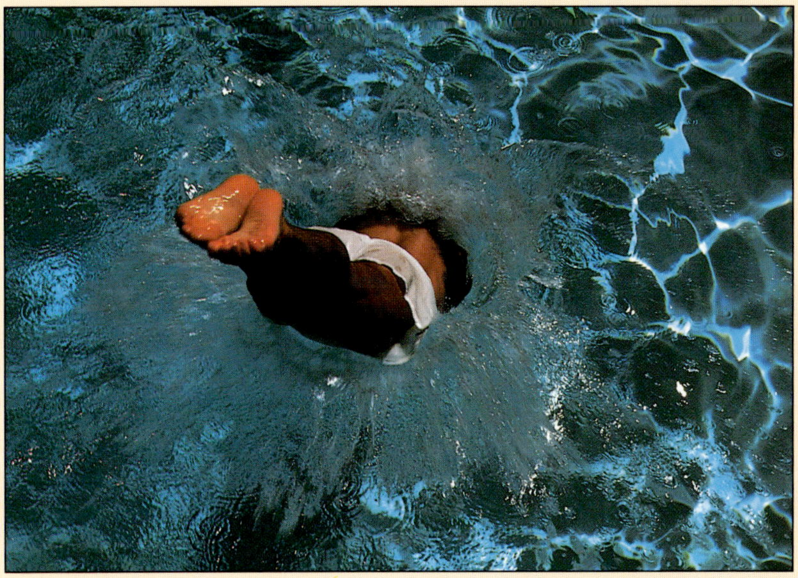

Nerves in your skin would quickly send messages to your brain to tell you which of these objects were comfortable to touch, and which were not.

There are five different ways of knowing things about the world around. They come to you through five senses: touch, taste, sight, sound and smell. Your senses are linked up to your brain through your nerves and quickly tell your brain what is happening around.

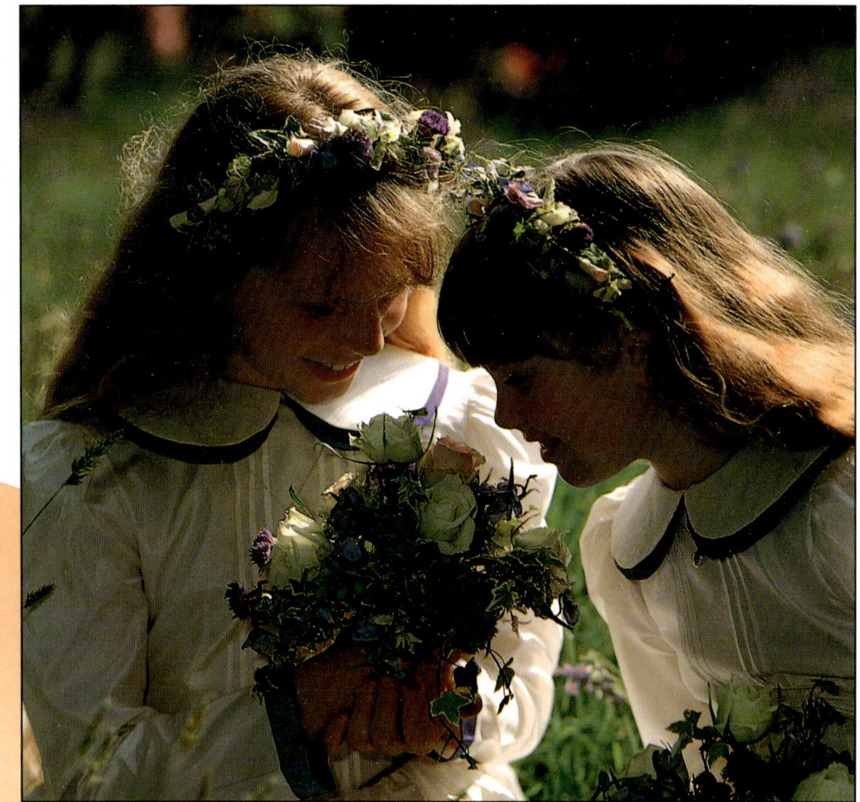

WHAT'S THAT SMELL?

You use your nose to smell things. Smells are caused by certain chemicals, which can travel through the air. When they reach a nerve in your nose, it sends a message to your brain explaining what the smell is like.

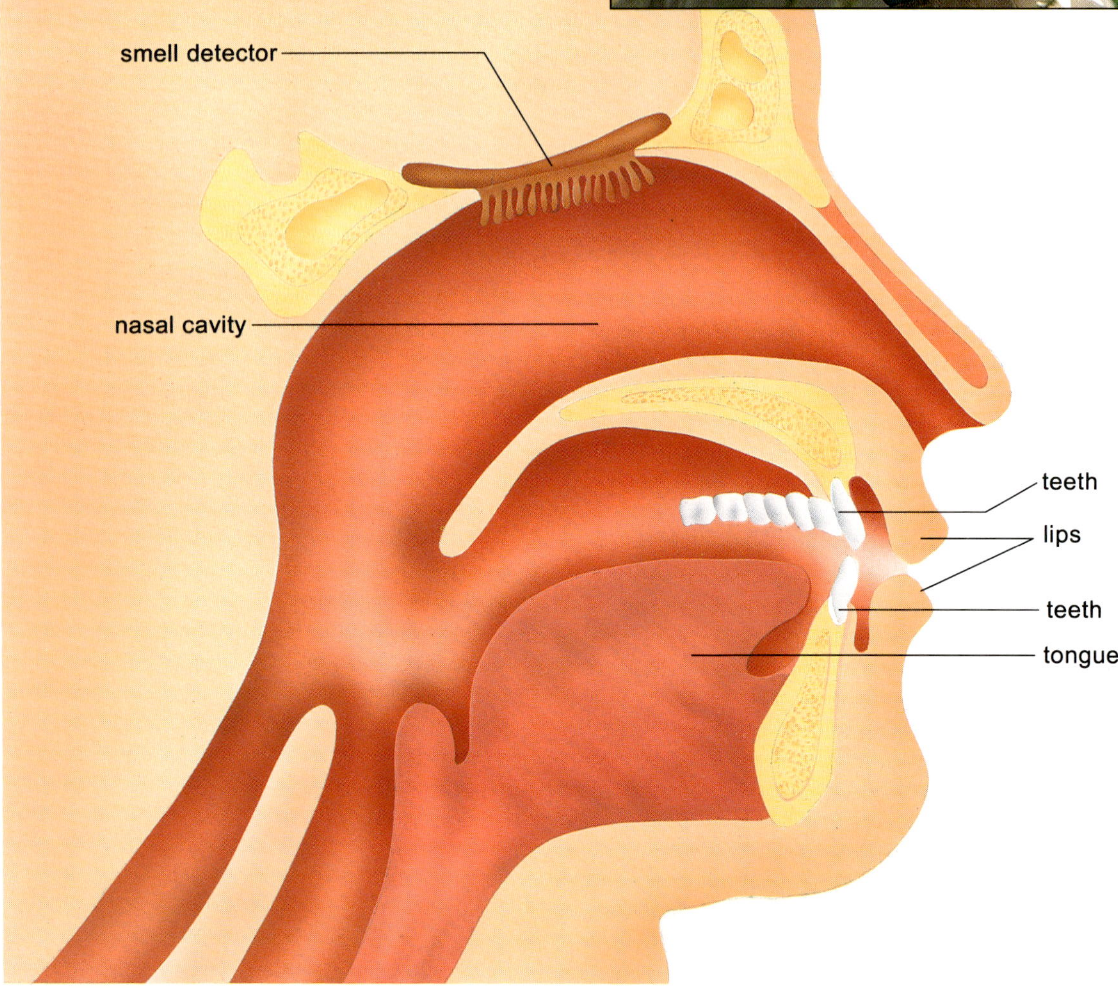

The smell of some flowers is so strong it travels for quite a distance around the plant. Other flowers have a weaker scent, and you have to get up close to smell them.

Your body's smell detector is in your nose. By sniffing in air near a smelly object, you also sniff in some of the chemicals that cause the smell. If you hold your nose you can't taste much, because the sense of smell is important in tasting flavours.

YUMMY!

What makes some food yummy and other food less so? It's what you feel about the taste! Thousands of tiny taste buds on your tongue tell your brain what food it likes.

Of course, people have very different ideas about what tastes they like.

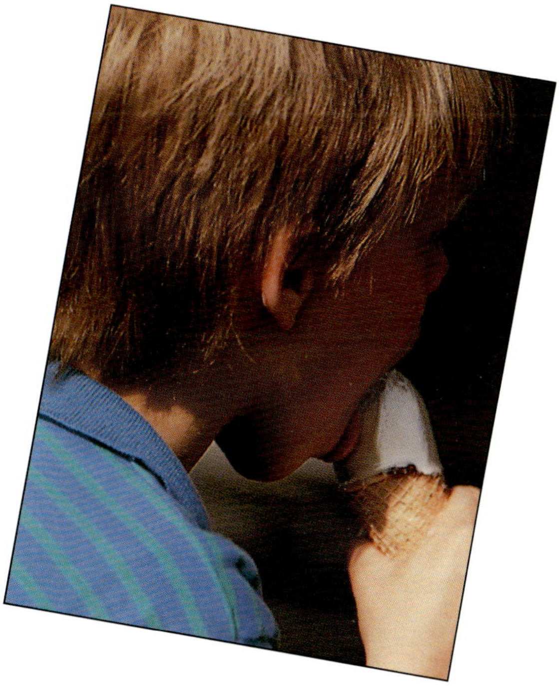

Taste buds can pick out the difference between sweet, sour, salt and bitter. Different areas of your tongue are sensitive to each of these four flavours.

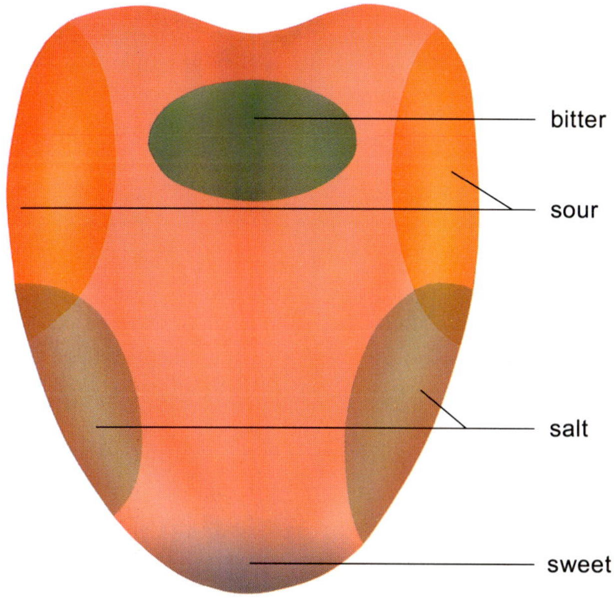

AT YOUR FINGERTIPS

The skin all over your body can feel things. The nerves in the skin enable you to pick out the difference between rough and smooth, hot and cold, wet and dry, and so on.

The fingertips are particularly sensitive. This helps your fingers to do all kinds of detailed work. The soles of your feet are usually a lot less sensitive, so you can walk around without noticing every detail of what you're treading on.

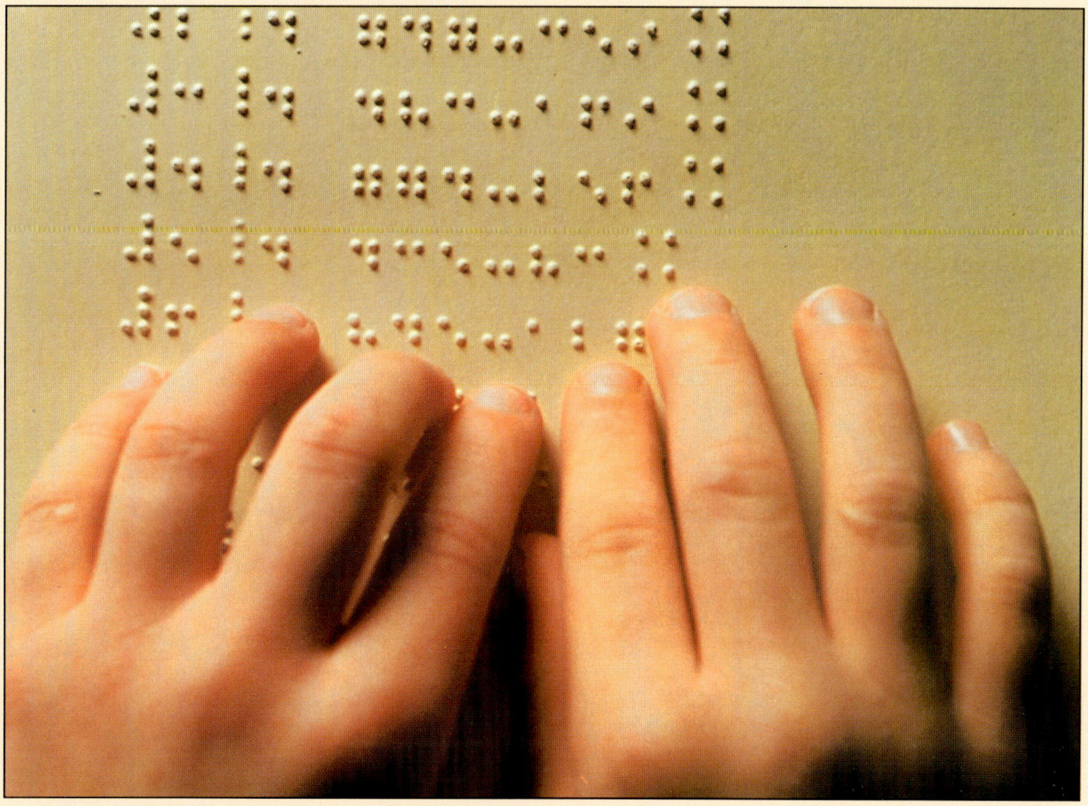

In this picture someone is using their fingertips to read the raised dots of the Braille alphabet.

SEE AND HEAR!

Of the five senses, sight and hearing probably make the most difference to people's lives, telling them a great deal about what is going on around them.

Blowing too hard on a recorder can make the notes go out of tune. People who want to play a musial instrument have to listen carefully to the sounds they are making.

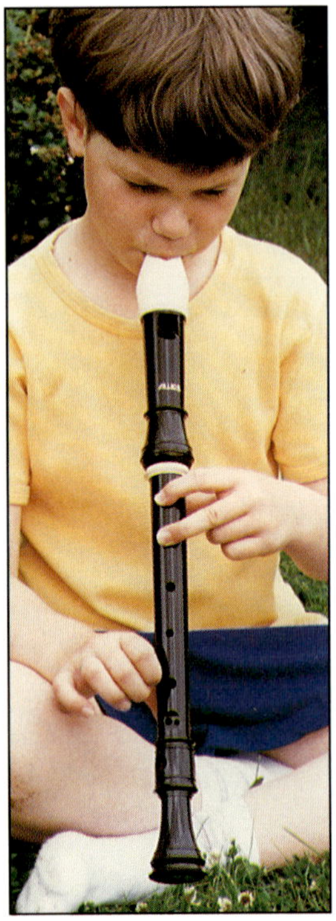

HEAR, HEAR

What you call your ears are only a part of the equipment your body has to hear sounds. The delicate shell-shapes on the side of a person's head collect sound. The bits which have hearing nerves in them are hidden away inside.

Sound is caused by vibrations, which shake the air in what are called sound waves. Your outer ear collects these and channels them down a tube so they strike a piece of stretched 'skin' called the ear-drum. This vibrates tiny bones inside, which set off more vibrations in the fluid in the inner ear. The vibrating fluid brushes against nerve cells, which send messages to the brain.

The brain learns to recognize many different sounds.

A cross-section through the ear.

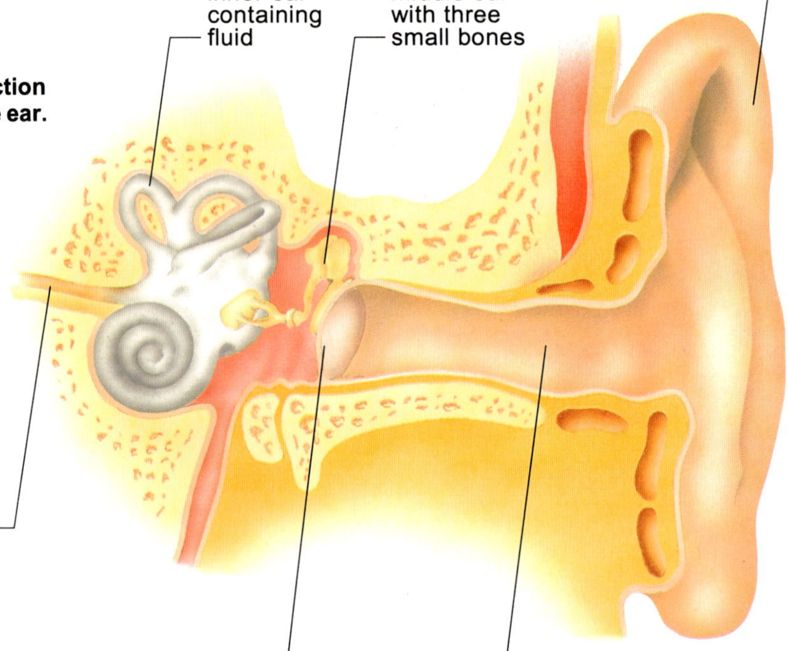

SPEAK UP!

Some people do not hear as well as others. A number of people find that they hear less well as they grow older. They may find it helpful to wear a hearing aid, a tiny instrument that can be fitted by the ear to amplify the sounds—to make them louder.

People who do not have any hearing from when they are tiny face a real challenge. They don't hear sounds, so they don't know how to make the sounds people use for speaking. It takes a lot of patient work for them to learn how to make sounds that *others* can hear and understand.

Some people who have no hearing prefer to communicate using a system of hand and arm signals called sign language.

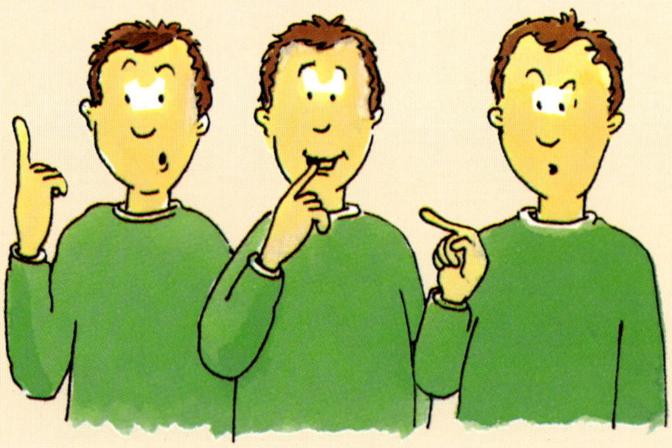

In one sign language these gestures mean 'Who told you?'

SEEING THE SIGHTS

When you look at something, your eye can tell you all kinds of things at the same time. It is able to tell whether the thing you are looking at is dark or light, what shape it is, what color it is, and what happens when it moves.

Rays of light travel from an object through to a lens near the front of your eye. This lens is operated by muscles that can adjust its shape so that it focuses the light onto the back of your eye, the retina. This is full of nerve cells that pass messages back to the brain. Your brain learns to make sense of many different objects.

The colored part of your eye is called the iris. It is a type of muscle. What you see as a black dot in the middle is the hole that lets the light through: the pupil. When you are in dim light, the iris contracts to make the pupil larger, which lets more light in. When you are in bright light, it relaxes to make the pupil smaller and let less light in.

The different parts of the eyeball, seen in cross-section. The eyeball is protected by the eye sockets of the skull.

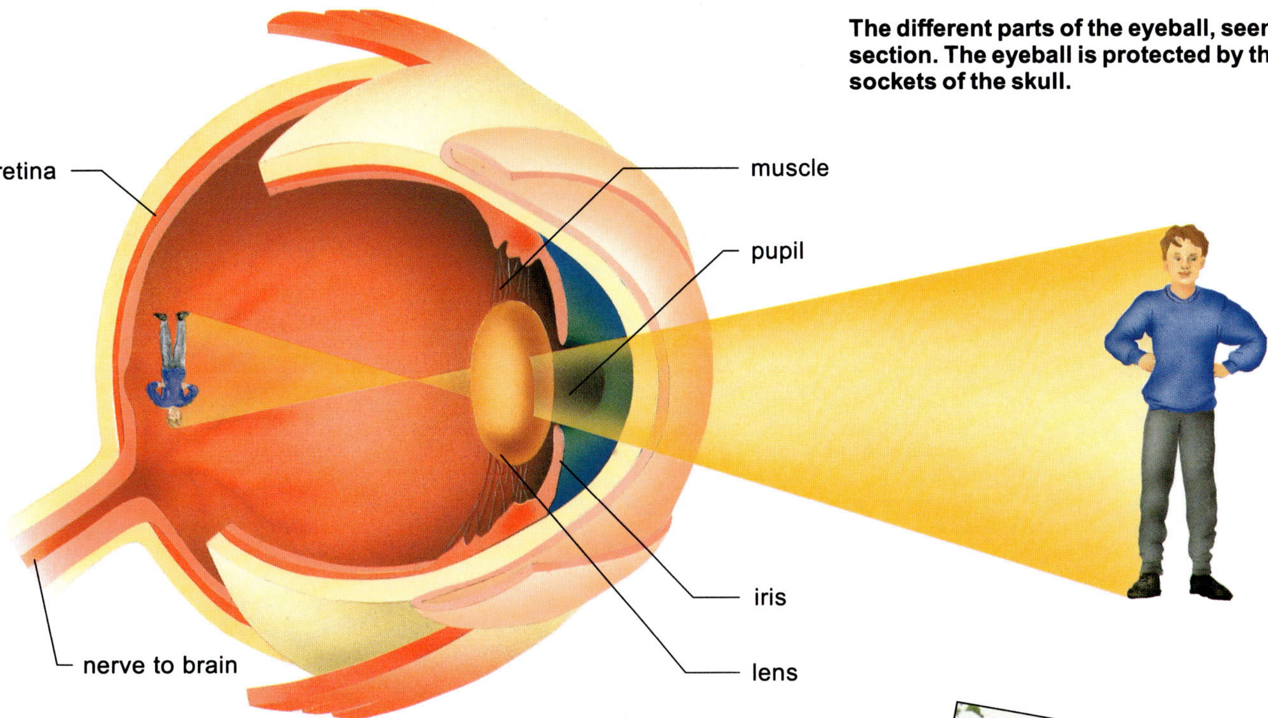

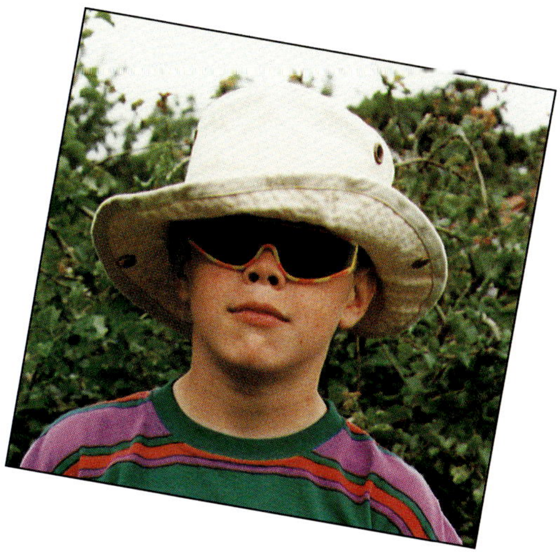

Bright sunlight can damage your eyes. This is uncomfortable at the time and can cause a thickening of the lens called a 'cataract' as you get older. Sunglasses help protect your eyes—as well as looking cool.

GETTING ABOUT

Getting about is a challenge for people who do not see well. Think how different it would be finding your way if you couldn't see the edge of the pavement, the road signs, the traffic, and so on.

People who don't see well have to learn new ways to get about. They may use a stick to help them feel what is ahead of them. Some people have guide dogs, which are trained to lead their owner safely around.

Some people find it helpful to wear spectacles. These have glass or plastic lenses that make it easier for the lens *in* the eye to focus light onto the retina. Without this clear focus, people may see some things as a bit of a blur rather than with clear, sharp edges.

TWENTY-FOUR HOUR PUMP—THE HEART

If you put your hand on the left side of your chest, you will feel a rhythmic beat. Hooray! Your heart's working.

The heart beats like this because it is pumping blood round the body. The blood acts like a transport system for the body, taking oxygen to all parts of the body. It also takes good things such as food to where it is needed, and carries out waste.

Although the heart isn't very big, it is very important. It has to keep beating all day, every day, for the body to go on working. A person whose heart stops beating for more than three minutes will probably die—unless they are kept alive on an artificial heart and lung machine.

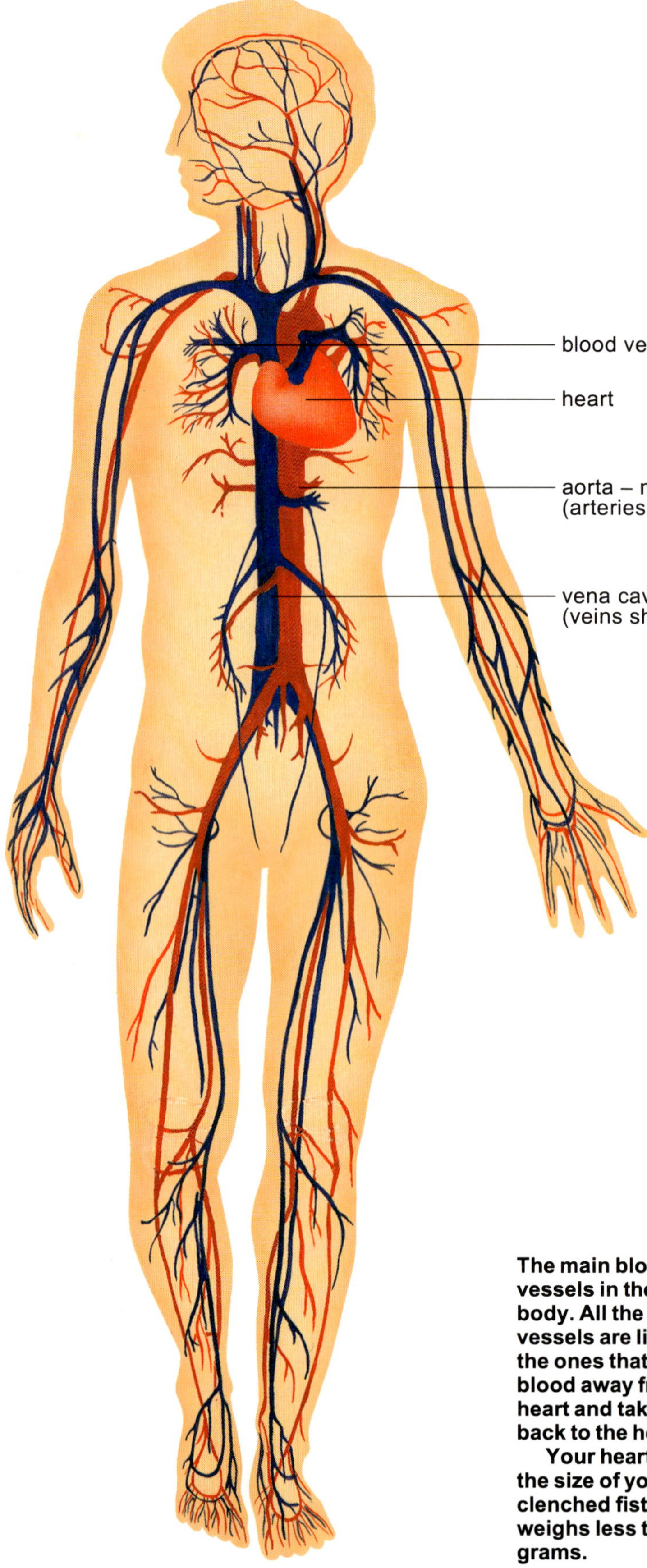

RECYCLING

The blood travels in tubes called arteries to get to the different parts of the body. It travels back to the heart in tubes called veins.

This network of tubes is rather like a tree. The veins and arteries are branches. Near the surface of the skin they have divided into lots of tiny tubes, like twigs. These are called capillaries.

The blood in the arteries is bright red because it has come from the lungs full of oxygen, to take to other parts of the body.

The blood in the veins is purplish-red because it carries only a small amount of oxygen. In its place is carbon dioxide—the gas the body puts back in the blood once it has used the oxygen. The veins carry the 'used' blood back to the heart and then the lungs to get rid of the carbon dioxide, which is breathed out. There, it takes in more oxygen that has been breathed in.

PUMP ACTION

The heart is very efficient. With every beat it pumps one cup of blood through your blood vessels. There are valves inside your heart to stop the blood running back, to make sure it goes in the right direction.

In one minute your heart can pump seven litres of blood round your body. When you are running or exercising hard, it can pump as much as fourteen litres round the body in one minute to get oxygen to all the parts of the body.

The main blood vessels in the human body. All the blood vessels are linked to the ones that carry blood away from the heart and take blood back to the heart.

Your heart is about the size of your clenched fist and weighs less than 200 grams.

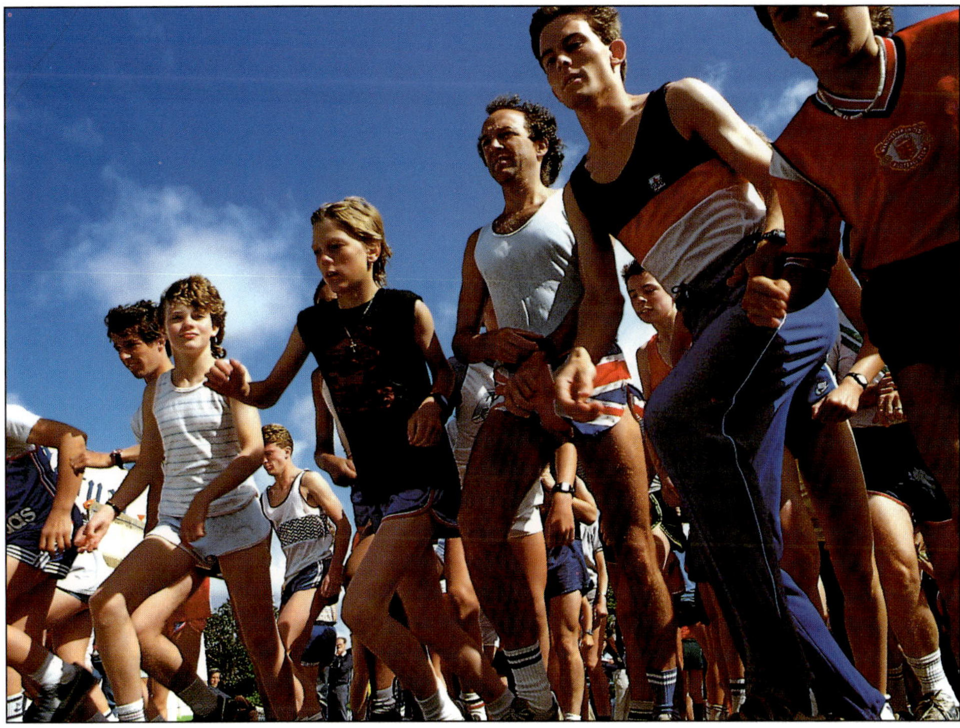

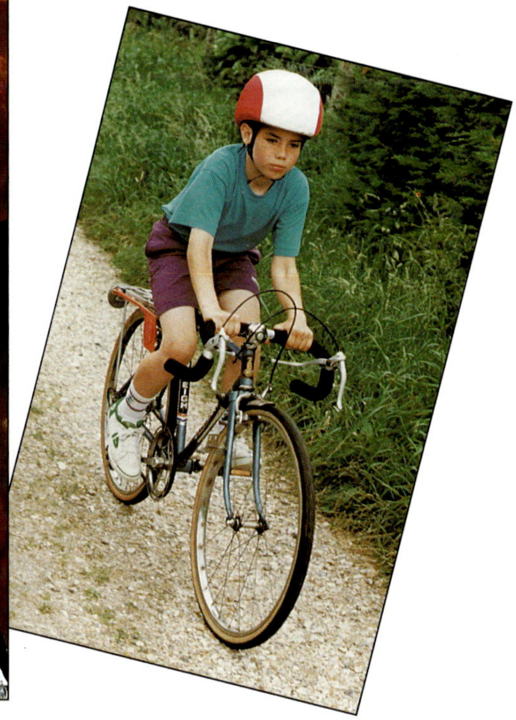

FIT FOR ANYTHING

You may have heard of aerobic exercises. These are strenuous exercises designed to make your heart work hard. People who do this kind of exercise carefully and regularly make their hearts stronger—and that allows them to run further and exercise harder.

Jogging, cycling and fast walking, as well as special dance routines, are all good aerobic exercises.

The blood in the arteries travels rather jerkily, as it is pushed further along with each heartbeat. The blood in veins flows more smoothly. Special valves act as one-way doors to stop the blood flowing backwards in them. You can see these as lumps on the veins of your hands or forearms.

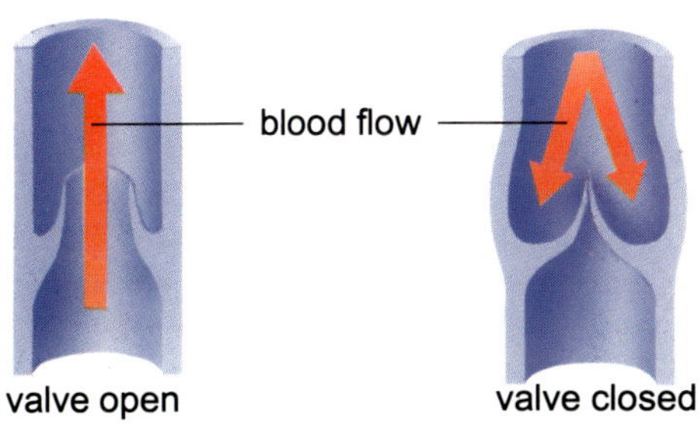

FINGER ON THE PULSE

There are places in your body where an artery is near the surface, and you can feel the jerky flow of the blood as your heart beats. These are called pulse points.

Feel your pulse

Try putting the tips of your two fingers on the inside of your wrist. Move these gently, pushing slightly, till you feel a gentle throb.

Or try putting two fingertips to one side of your neck, at the top where it joins the chin. This pulse is stronger.

Count the number of beats. You will find that your heart beats at different rates depending on what you have been doing. It is easiest to count the beats for 10 seconds, and multiply the result by six to get the rate per minute.

Compare yourself with these results:

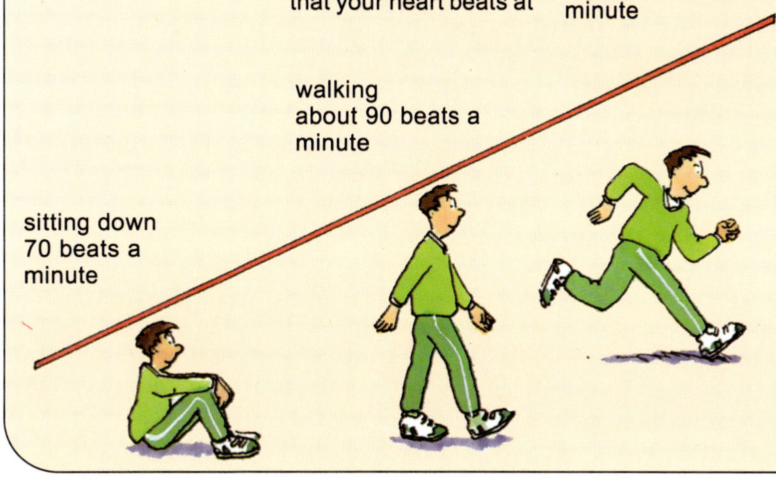
running
about 110 beats a minute
walking
about 90 beats a minute
sitting down
70 beats a minute

EXPRESS TRANSPORT SYSTEM—BLOOD

The blood pumping round your body is a busy transport system carrying a lot of traffic. It is a liquid that carries oxygen, food, chemical messengers and waste products from one part of the body to another through the blood vessels.

WHAT COLOUR IS BLOOD?

If you look at your blood under a microscope, you will see it is made of a yellowish fluid called plasma. Dotted around are some large, shapeless white blood cells. The fluid is teeming with clumps of red blood cells that look like miniature flying saucers. These make blood look red.

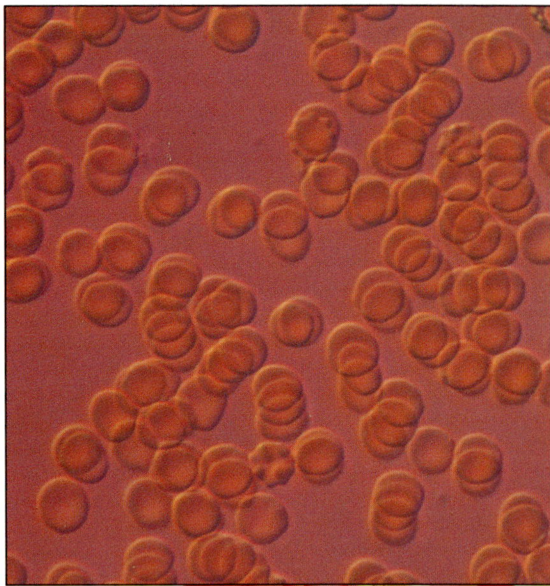

WHAT YOU DON'T SEE

There are lots of things in blood you can't see. Here are some of them:

- Oxygen. This is in the air you breathe in. All parts of the body need it to stay alive.
- Waste products, to be got rid of. One of these is carbon dioxide, which is in the air you breathe out.
- Food. The blood carries the goodness of food to the parts of your body that need it.
- Hormones. These are special chemical messengers. They whizz around at high speed from one part of your body to another, telling your body what to do and what not to do.

For example, some hormones control the speed at which you grow—not too fast, and not too slow.

Others make sure that if you are a boy, your body develops as a boy's should. If you are a girl, you develop as a girl should.

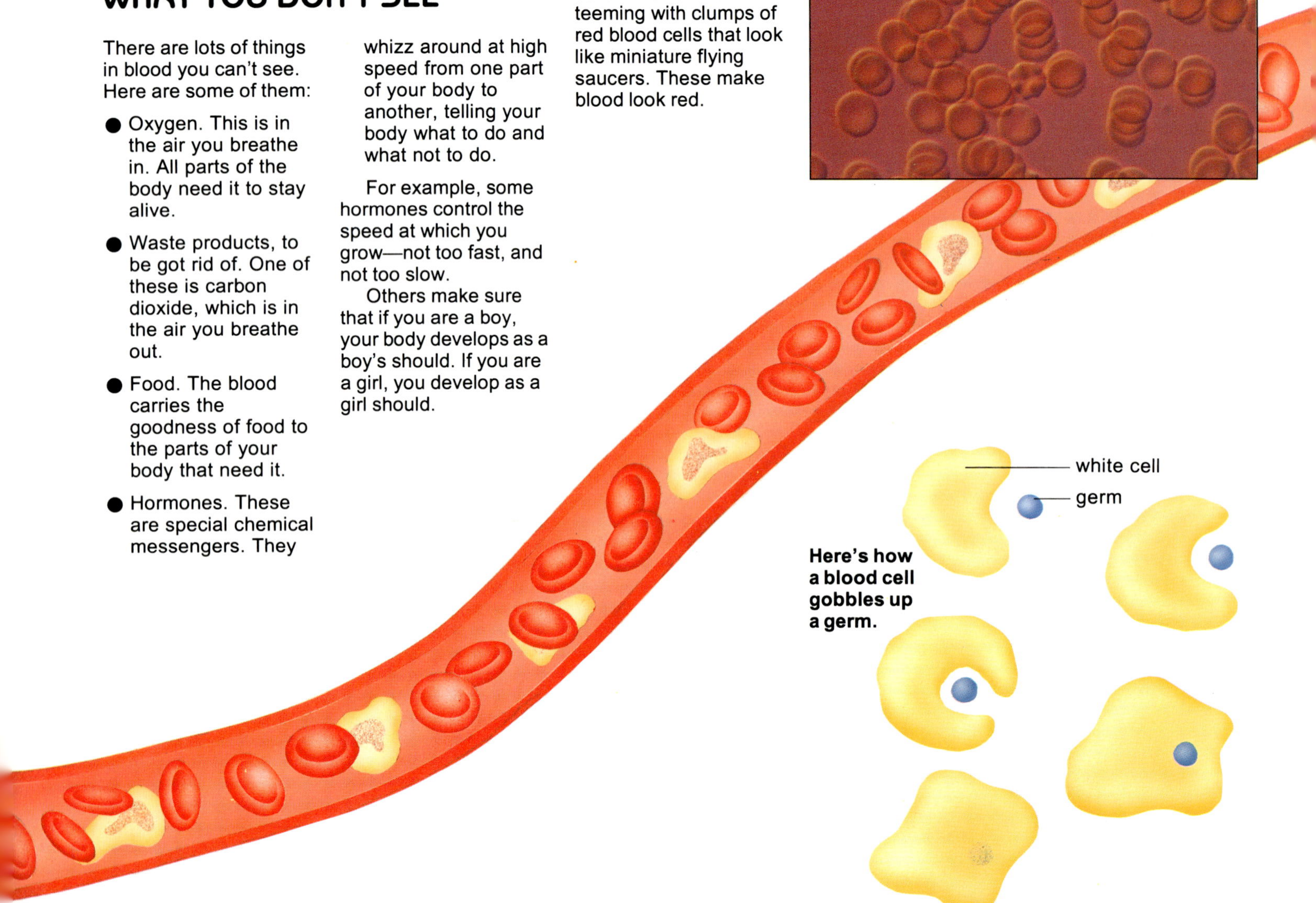

Here's how a blood cell gobbles up a germ.

RED CELLS AT WORK

The red blood cells grab hold of oxygen and rush it to the parts of your body that need it. That is how each part of the body has the energy it needs to do its work.

Human bodies have been designed to make sure that every part works together. Vital parts such as the brain and heart have priority for blood supplies because they need to work all the time.

WHITE CELLS AT WORK

White blood cells are important in battling against germs. Sometimes they massacre germs and carry them out of harm's way. At other times they shoot out antibodies which paralyse or kill the germs.

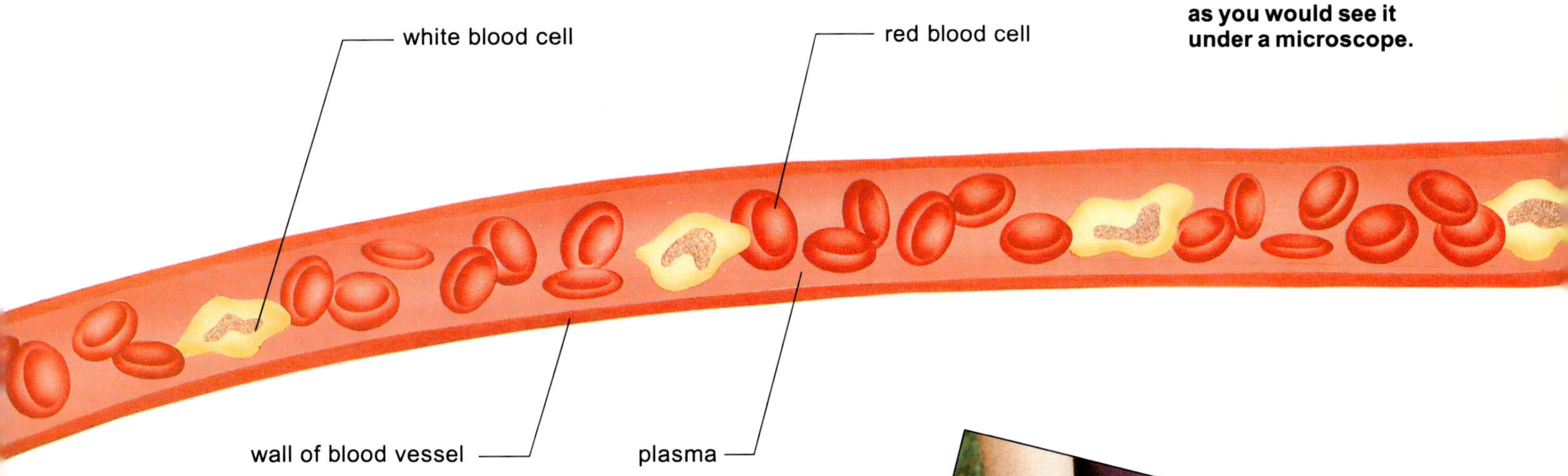

A blood vessel drawn as you would see it under a microscope.

HELP—I'M BLEEDING

When your nose bleeds or you cut yourself, the bleeding usually stops without anyone doing anything.

If you cut yourself, the tiny blood vessels begin to close up as soon as they have been damaged. Then special agents in the blood, called clotting factors, do their work. They come from the plasma and from the red blood cells and platelets (tiny bits of cells). When they are all blended together they form a tough clot that stops blood from getting out and germs from getting in. A scab is a dried-out blood clot.

If you pick a scab then you dislodge everything and the bleeding starts again.

If you cut a vein or an artery it is more difficult to get the bleeding to stop. The edges of the vein or artery need to be brought close together so they can begin to heal.

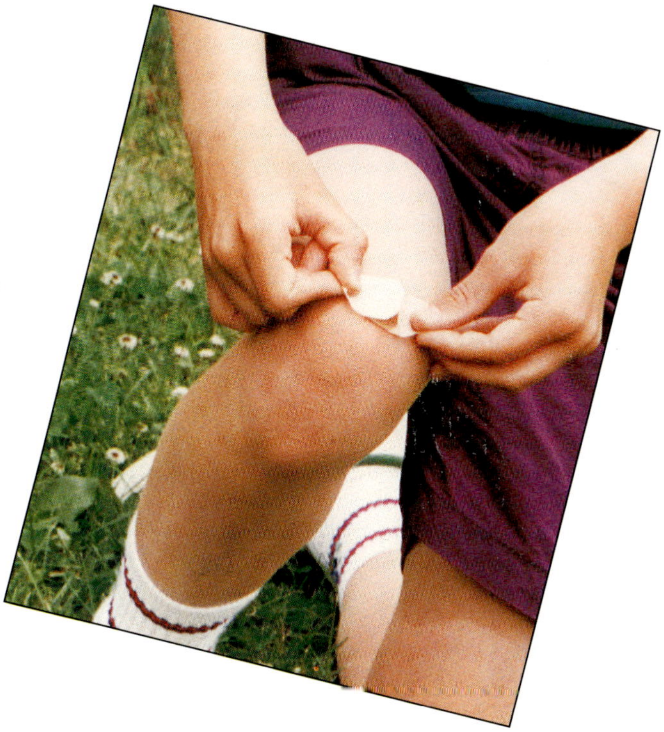

The stages in healing

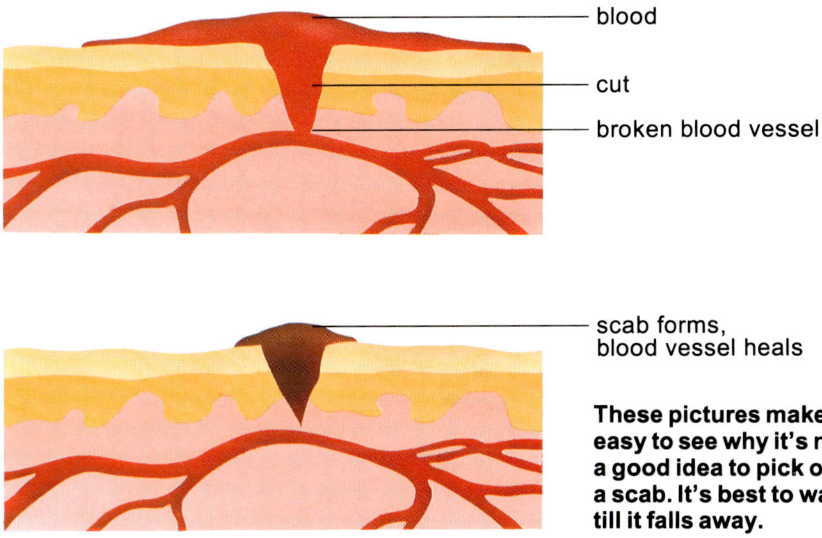

These pictures make it easy to see why it's not a good idea to pick off a scab. It's best to wait till it falls away.

First Aid Tips

- Keep the wound clean. It's a good idea to wash it in clean water.
- Stop the bleeding. Pressing hard on a cut helps stop the bleeding.
- Let the wound heal. Small cuts don't need a bandage. Once they have scabbed over, however, you may want to wear a light bandage to stop the scabs from getting knocked.
- Always ask a grown-up to check that a cut is all right, and always ask for help to treat a large wound.
- Try never to touch someone else's blood. Ask a grown-up to help if someone else has an accident.

SPRING CLEANERS—LUNGS

Can you hold your breath? You certainly have to hold it for a few seconds when you put your head under water to swim. But after a few seconds you have to come to the surface. Then you gasp out your breath, and gulp in fresh air.

Perhaps you can hold your breath for what seems like a long time. But people never really stop breathing until they die. A person needs to breathe, because the air supplies their blood with oxygen, the gas that the body needs for life.

As soon as a baby is born it yells and then starts to breathe for the first time, taking fresh air down the windpipe to the lungs. A person then goes on breathing for the rest of their life.

When a person breathes out air underwater it rises to the surface as bubbles.

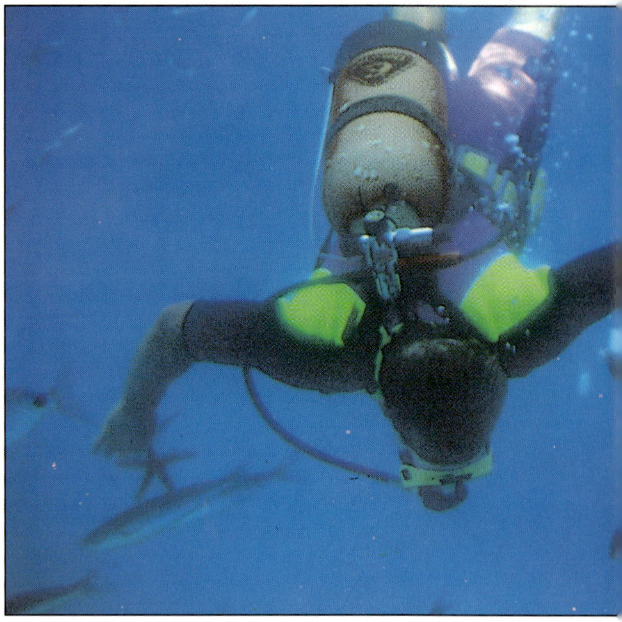

You have two lungs, one on each side of your chest. When you breathe, you can feel your chest going in and out. In your lungs is a complicated system of passage-ways, which branch rather like trees: the main 'trunk' tube divides into 'branch' tubes, and those branch into 'twig' tubes . . . and so on many times. This cross-section only shows the main divisions.

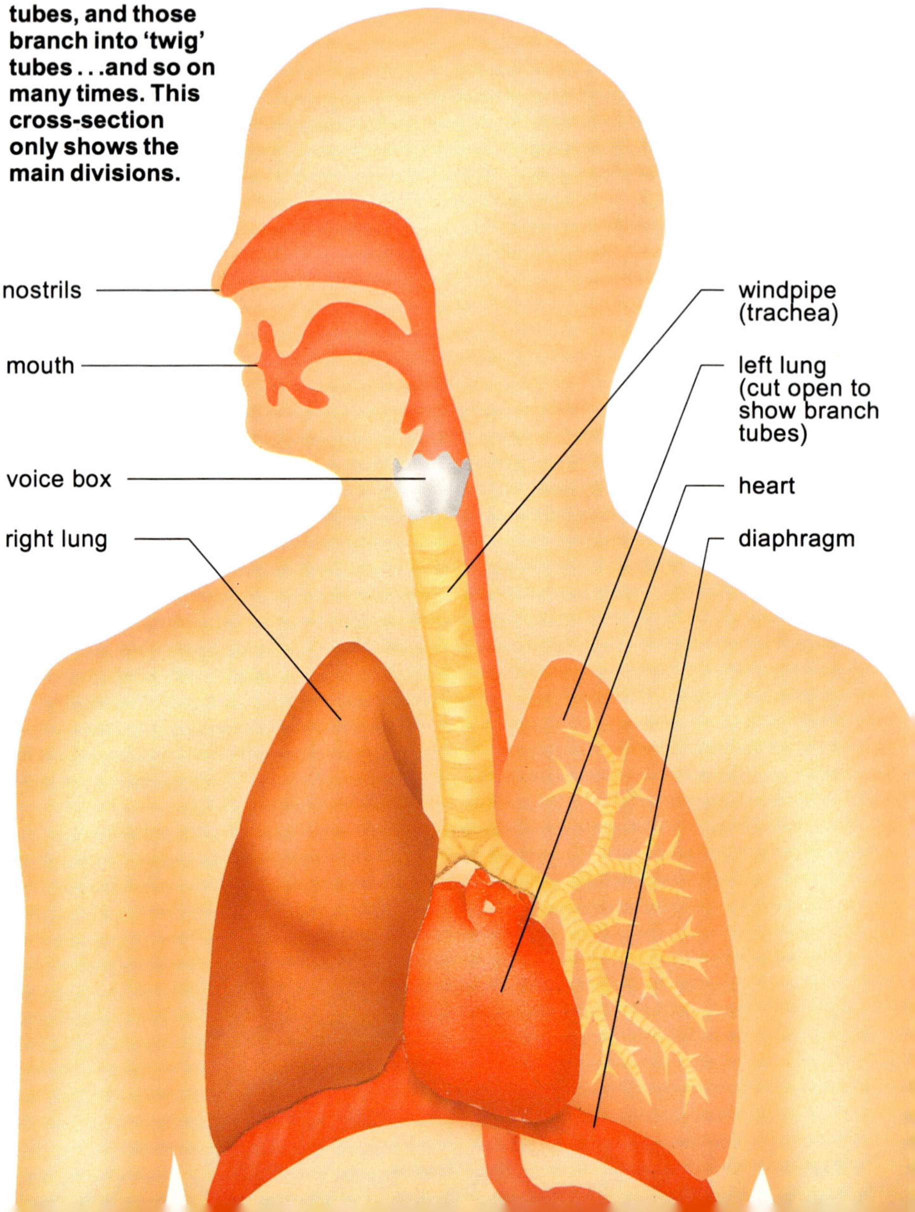

ALL CHANGE

The air you breathe in contains quite a lot of oxygen. Blood comes to the lungs and takes this oxygen round the body.

The blood also brings back the 'used up' gas—a different sort, called carbon dioxide.

I'M PUFFED!

When you exercise, your body needs extra oxygen.

Your heart beats fast to get blood round your body as quickly as possible. And you have to breathe fast to supply your blood with extra oxygen, and to breathe out the carbon dioxide that is made when that oxygen is used up.

That can leave you panting for air.

TAKE A DEEP BREATH

When you breathe in, your lungs get bigger, and when you breathe out they get smaller as all the air is pushed out.

Breathe in deeply and measure round your chest. Then breathe out, and measure it again. If you are very fit there will be 3 to 5 centimetres difference between the two measurements.

Taking regular exercise that makes your heart beat faster is the way to get fit. Then you'll have lots of energy for all the things you want to do!

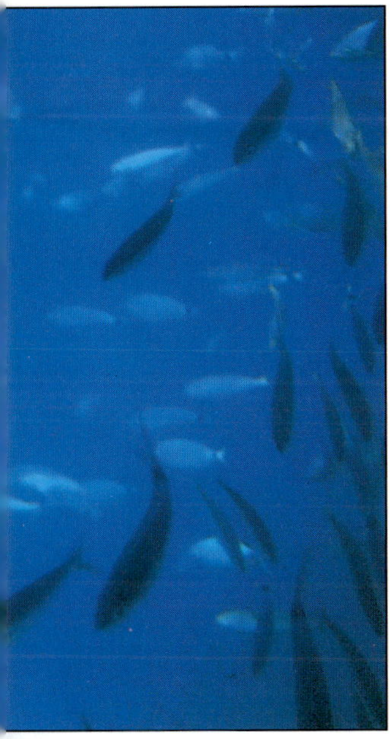

HIC!

When you hiccup you breathe in and out sharply and quickly. After each breath your voice-box closes with a snap and that makes you go 'hic'.

There are lots of different reasons why you hiccup. If you can't stop hiccuping for several days then it's worth going to see a doctor, to find out if something needs to be put right. But mostly it doesn't matter.

Sometimes you can stop hiccups by getting a cup full of water and then drinking from it by bending over the cup, and sipping the water from the wrong side of the cup.

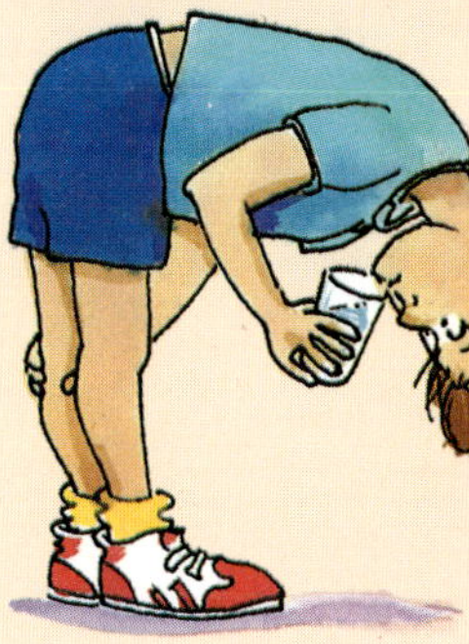

WHAT A YAWN!

When you yawn you are usually feeling tired or sleepy.

You yawn because, without your knowing it, your brain tells your lungs to help you wake up. You breathe very deeply without thinking about it first. This pulls extra air into your lungs to freshen them which helps you wake up.

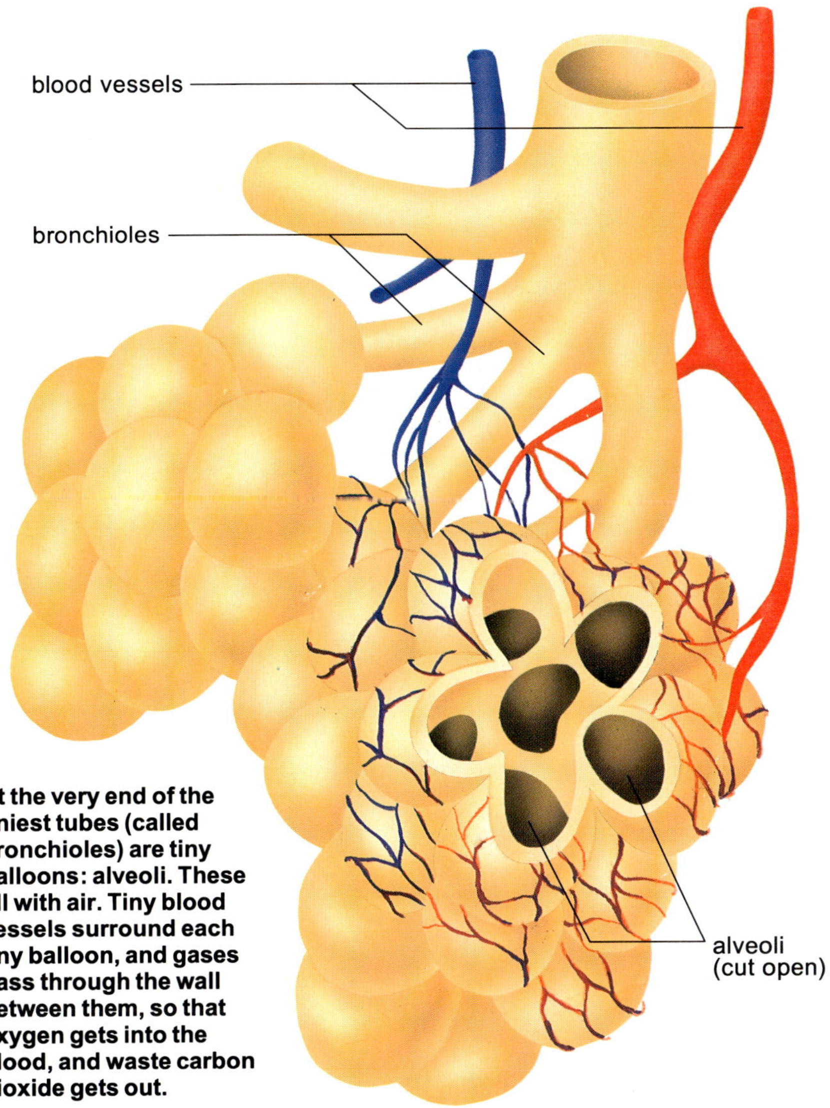

At the very end of the tiniest tubes (called bronchioles) are tiny balloons: alveoli. These fill with air. Tiny blood vessels surround each tiny balloon, and gases pass through the wall between them, so that oxygen gets into the blood, and waste carbon dioxide gets out.

SPEAK UP

To speak or sing, you have to push air from your lungs out past the vocal cords and through your nose and mouth. The muscles of the vocal cords can change length—short to make high notes, long for low notes. People make vowels (like ooh and aah) by changing the shape of their mouths—try it! Lips and teeth make the consonents, such as t and p. The harder you push air out, the louder the sound.

voice box

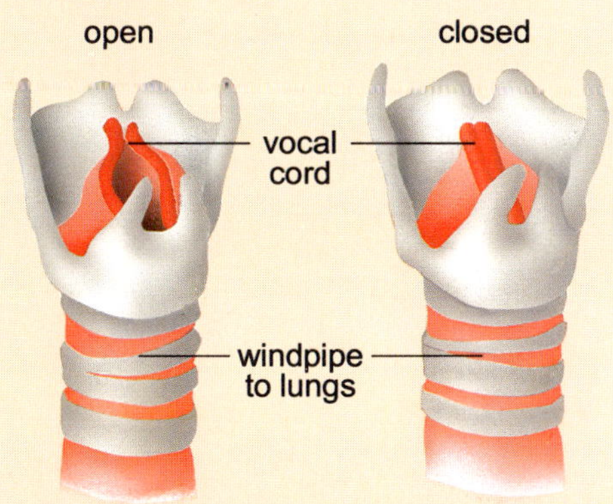

If you pluck strings of different lengths on a musical instrument they make different notes. You make different sounds by changing the length of your vocal cords, which are in the voice box.

FOOD PROCESSING—STOMACH AND INTESTINES

The body must have food to supply it with energy—fuel for all the different things the body does.

Food also provides other things the body needs to grow: for making new cells, for example, so that you grow strong and stay healthy.

But the body has some hard work to do to break the food down so it can use it in these different ways. This breaking-down process is called digestion. The stomach and intestines are the digestive system—the food processing unit of your body.

The digestive system

You use your tongue and teeth to chew food in your mouth.

The chewed food goes down a tube called the oesophagus.

In the stomach special chemicals act on the food, making it softer and more liquid.

When the food is ready, a valve at the end of the stomach lets it into the intestine.

In the intestine, different chemicals break the food down even more. The goodness is taken out, and travels in the blood to where it is needed.

The appendix is a little blind-ended tube that sometimes gets blocked and infected causing appendicitis, which needs an operation. Humans don't need an appendix!

The waste food goes right down to the end of the intestines. It comes out of the body through the anus when you go to the toilet.

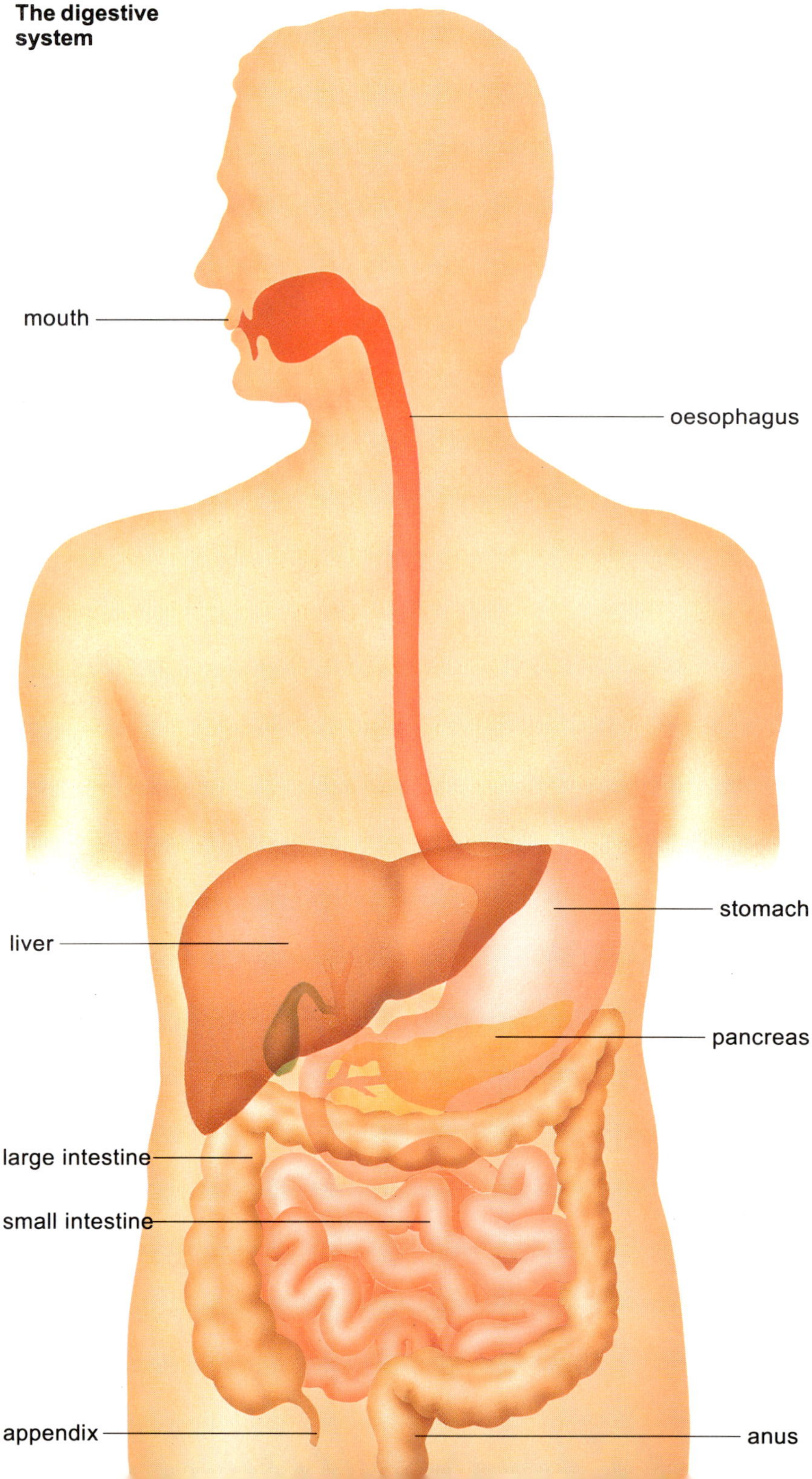

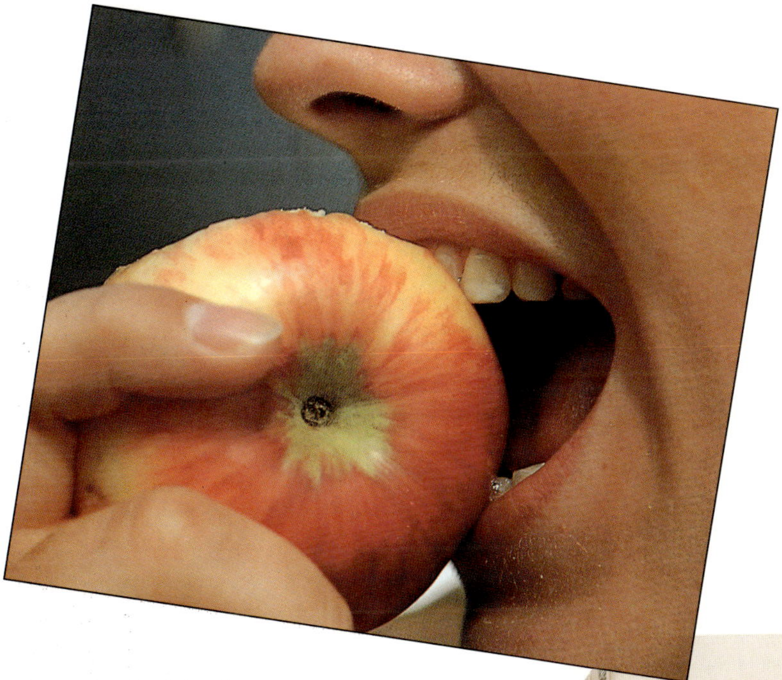

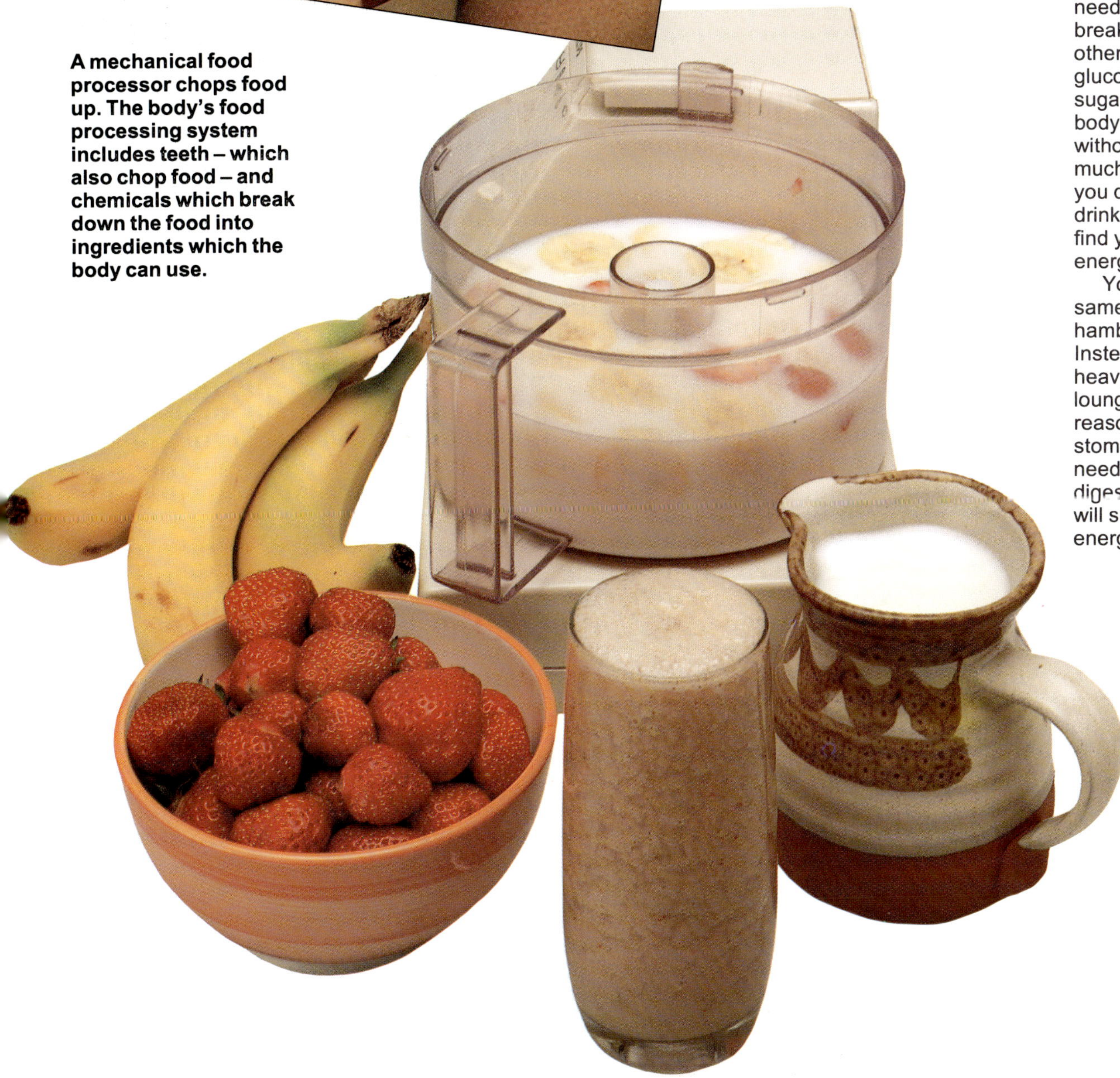

A mechanical food processor chops food up. The body's food processing system includes teeth – which also chop food – and chemicals which break down the food into ingredients which the body can use.

THE WRONG WAY

Food doesn't usually move backwards, as there are valves which act like one-way doors to stop this. But if there is something wrong, you may vomit. What happens is that your stomach squeezes backwards, propelling part-digested food back into your mouth.

A QUICK BURST OF ENERGY

Some foods do not need much work to break them down; others need a lot. A glucose drink contains sugar in a form your body can use quickly without having to do much to it. So, when you drink a glucose drink, you will probably find you have a burst of energy.

You won't get the same result if you eat a hamburger and chips. Instead, you may feel heavy and prefer to lounge around. The reason is that your stomach and intestines need to work hard to digest the food before it will supply you with energy.

FOOD, GLORIOUS FOOD

Eating food is fun. You'd probably like to have your favourite food at every meal. But one sort of food isn't enough. You need a balance of the right foods to provide your body with what it needs.

The things that foods provide can be sorted into different groups. To stay healthy, you need to have some from each group every day.

As well, you need to make sure that your food contains a range of vitamins, which help your body grow properly. Your body cannot store vitamins and it can't manufacture most of them, so you must be sure to eat food that has them in.

FOOD GROUPS

- Proteins—for growth and repair. Found in fish, eggs, meat, milk, cheese, cereals, nuts, beans, lentils, peas.

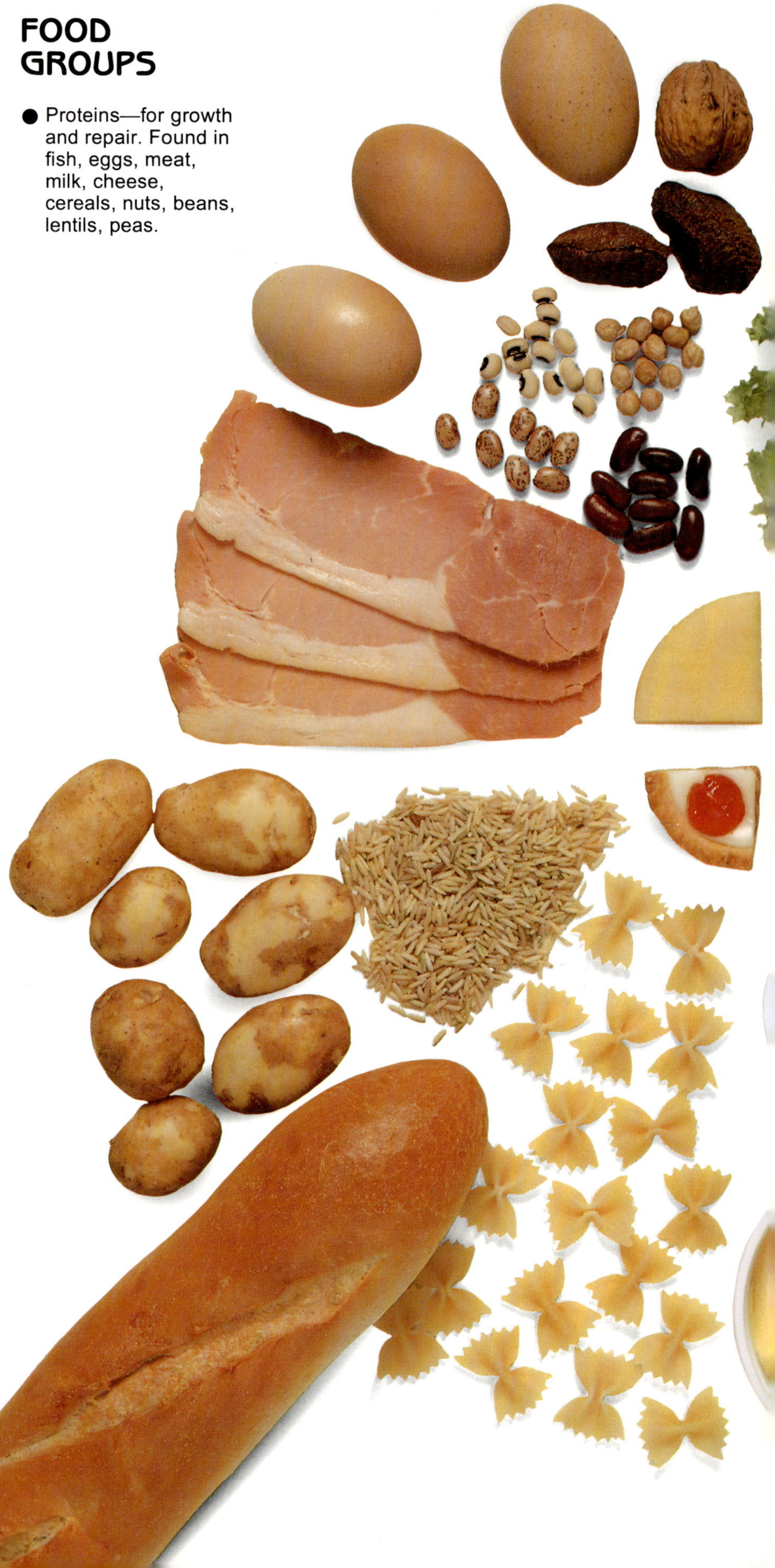

There are lots of different vitamins. They are often called after letters of the alphabet. Here are a few:

A—found in fruit, yellow vegetables. People need vitamin A to see well.

B—found in eggs, meat, whole wheat, oats, yeast. Vitamin B1 keeps nerves working. There are lots of different B vitamins.

C—found in fruit, especially oranges. Vitamin C keeps skin and gums healthy.

D—found in margarine, oily fish. Vitamin D helps keep bones strong.

- Carbohydrates—for energy. Found in potatoes, pasta, rice, bread, cereals, root vegetables, sugar, biscuits, cakes.

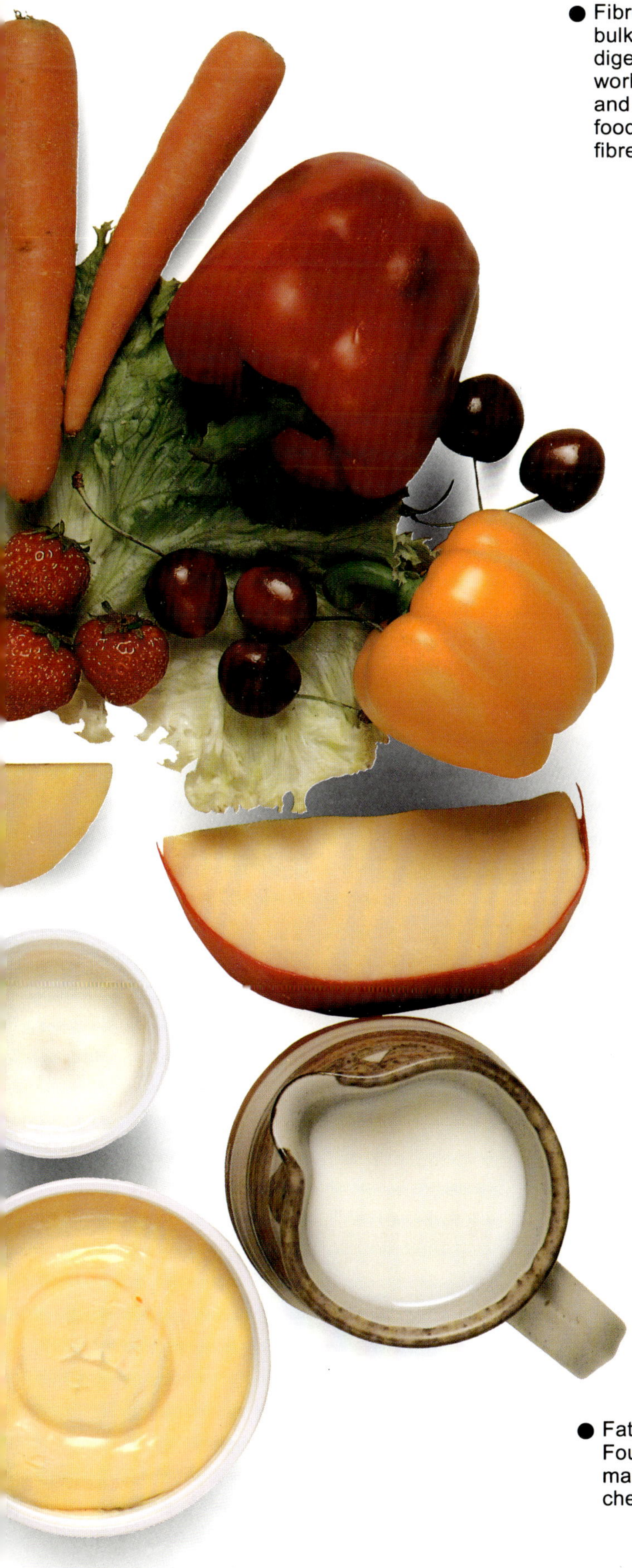

- Fibre—provides the bulk that helps your digestive system to work. Vegetables and whole-grain foods have a lot of fibre.

FOOD STORES

Your body stores any food that it doesn't need to use straight away, ready for when you might need it. Different kinds of food are stored in different places. Some food is stored in the fat layers of your body.

This store of fat is useful to provide extra energy if you need it. That's really important, because everybody needs energy, even if they don't do anything really active: some energy is still needed to keep your heart beating and your lungs working, as well as lots of other things your body does automatically. If you have to go without food, your body can use some of its energy store to keep all these things happening.

If the fat is used, the person looks thinner. If people regularly eat more food than they need for energy, they may get fatter. To be healthy, you need to keep a good balance between how much food you eat and how much energy you use.

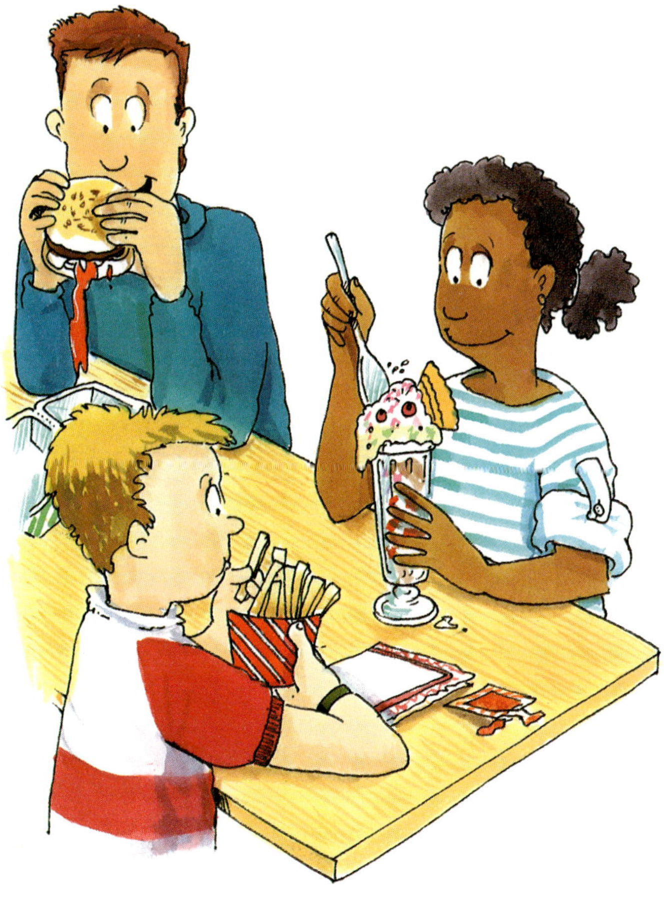

Crisps, sweets, fizzy drinks . . . junk food such as this fills you up with fats and carbohydrates (mainly in the form of sugar). Only having foods of one 'food type' can leave people starved of the nutrients they need.

- Fats—for energy. Found in butter, margarine, oils, milk, cheese.

THE BODY'S WASTE DISPOSAL UNITS—KIDNEYS

As your cells and tissues work, they make waste stuff which must be removed or you will die.

Your blood carries carbon dioxide waste to the lungs. Other waste goes to your kidneys.

You have two kidneys lying at the back of you, just below the bottom of your chest. Each is quite small—about 10 centimetres long—and weighs about 150 grams. The kidneys are the body's filter system, for taking out waste products.

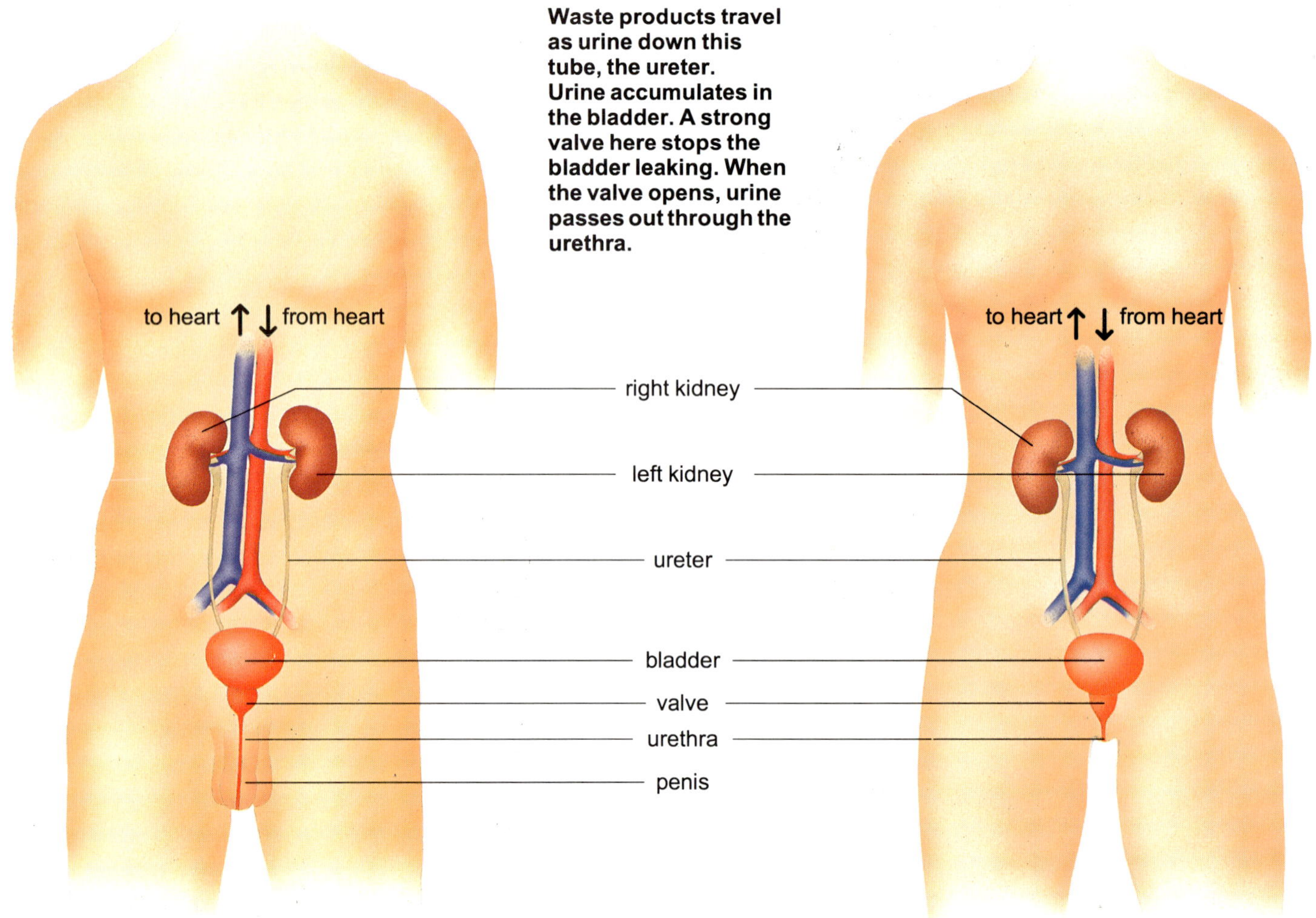

TOILET TROUBLE

Babies aren't able to decide when to 'go to the toilet'—and when not to. They begin to learn this in the first years of life, usually after they can walk and talk. Often, parents will teach them to use their own little toilet: a potty!

Sometimes older children wet their pants, perhaps because they are excited, tired or ill. Some wet their beds when they are asleep. Some people take longer to grow out of bedwetting than others, and some need help learning to stop.

Sometimes adults 'leak' when they don't want to. This is called incontinence and may be due to illness or old age, or to some damage to the muscles and valves that stop the bladder leaking. The problem can often be fixed. If it can't, people can wear pads to absorb the moisture, which they then throw away.

THE FILTER SYSTEM

A filter is a barrier that lets some things through and not others. The kidneys are the body's filters. As blood passes through them, it keeps back the waste products in it and lets the cleaned blood through.

Then the waste products travel out from each kidney as urine. This passes down a tube to your bladder, at the bottom of your tummy.

Your bladder has a strong valve to it. This stops your urine from leaking out all the time. When you go to the toilet, the valve relaxes and opens so that urine is allowed out.

DID YOU KNOW?

Kidneys are capable of doing far more work than they usually do. This means that a person can stay fit and alive with only one kidney.

If someone's kidneys have stopped working, there is a problem of how to filter the waste out of their body. One way is to link them up to a machine that filters their blood. Another is to give them someone else's kidney, if a suitable donor can be found.

Nowadays surgeons are able to do tests to find out if a certain kidney is suitable for a person whose kidneys have stopped working. If it is, they can do an operation to take the kidney from the donor and put it perfectly in place in the person who needs a working kidney.

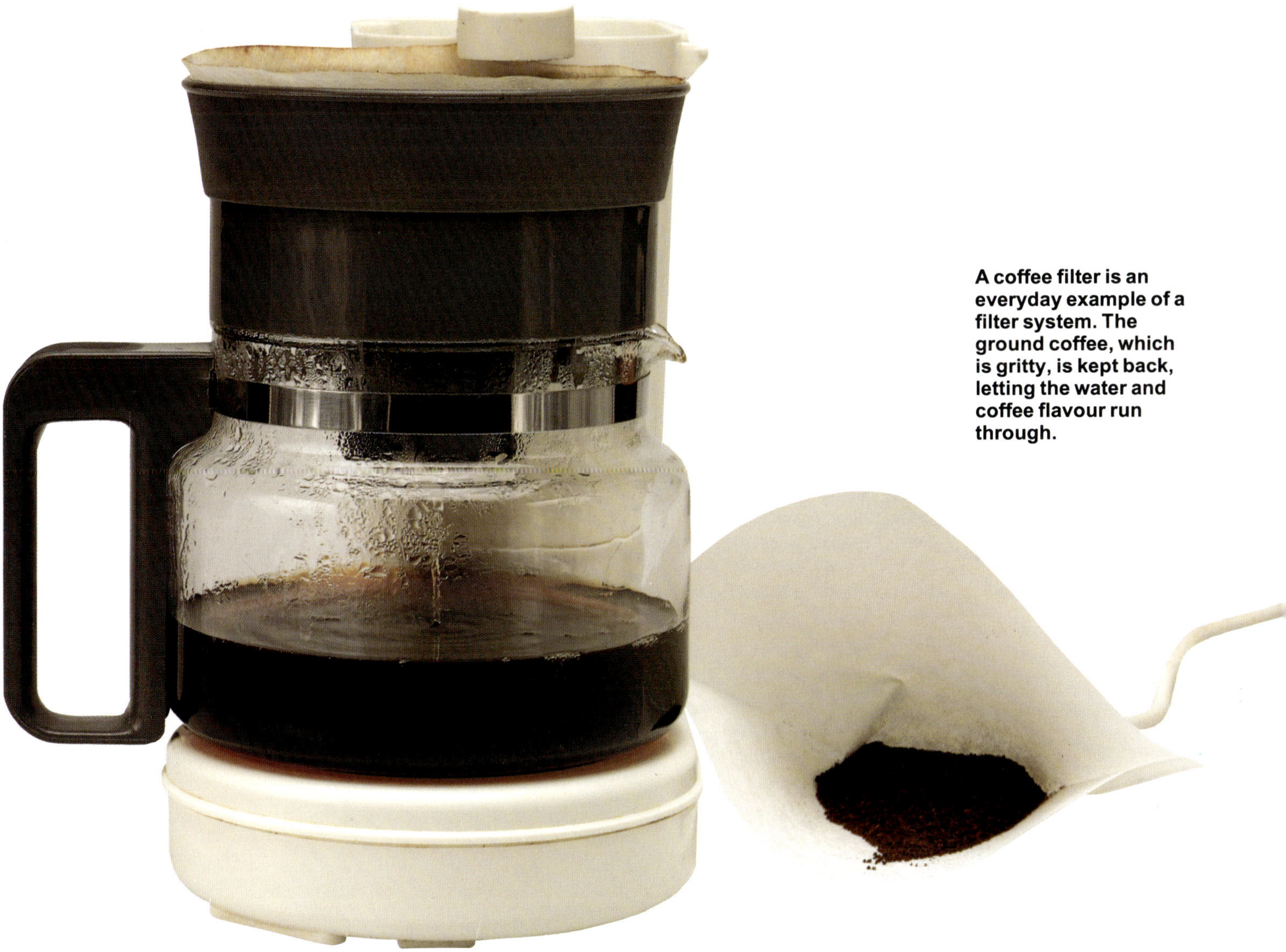

A coffee filter is an everyday example of a filter system. The ground coffee, which is gritty, is kept back, letting the water and coffee flavour run through.

KEEPING YOU STRAIGHT—BONES

Your body is built around a framework of bones, which are joined to one another to make you the shape you are. This framework is called the skeleton.

Some bones hold you in shape. Your arms and legs are shaped around long, straightish bones. Your backbone holds your body in a line. It is made of a column of small bones, one on top of the other. These little bones are called vertebrae, and the whole column is called the spine.

Other bones give protection as well as shape. They surround delicate organs so they do not get bruised or squashed. The brain is fragile, so it is kept safe inside the head bone, the skull, which acts as its safety helmet. The lungs and heart are protected by the ribcage.

Bones are very tough. They are full of calcium—which is made into a cement which fills up the spaces between the living bone cells. Bones that do not have enough calcium bend more easily than they should.

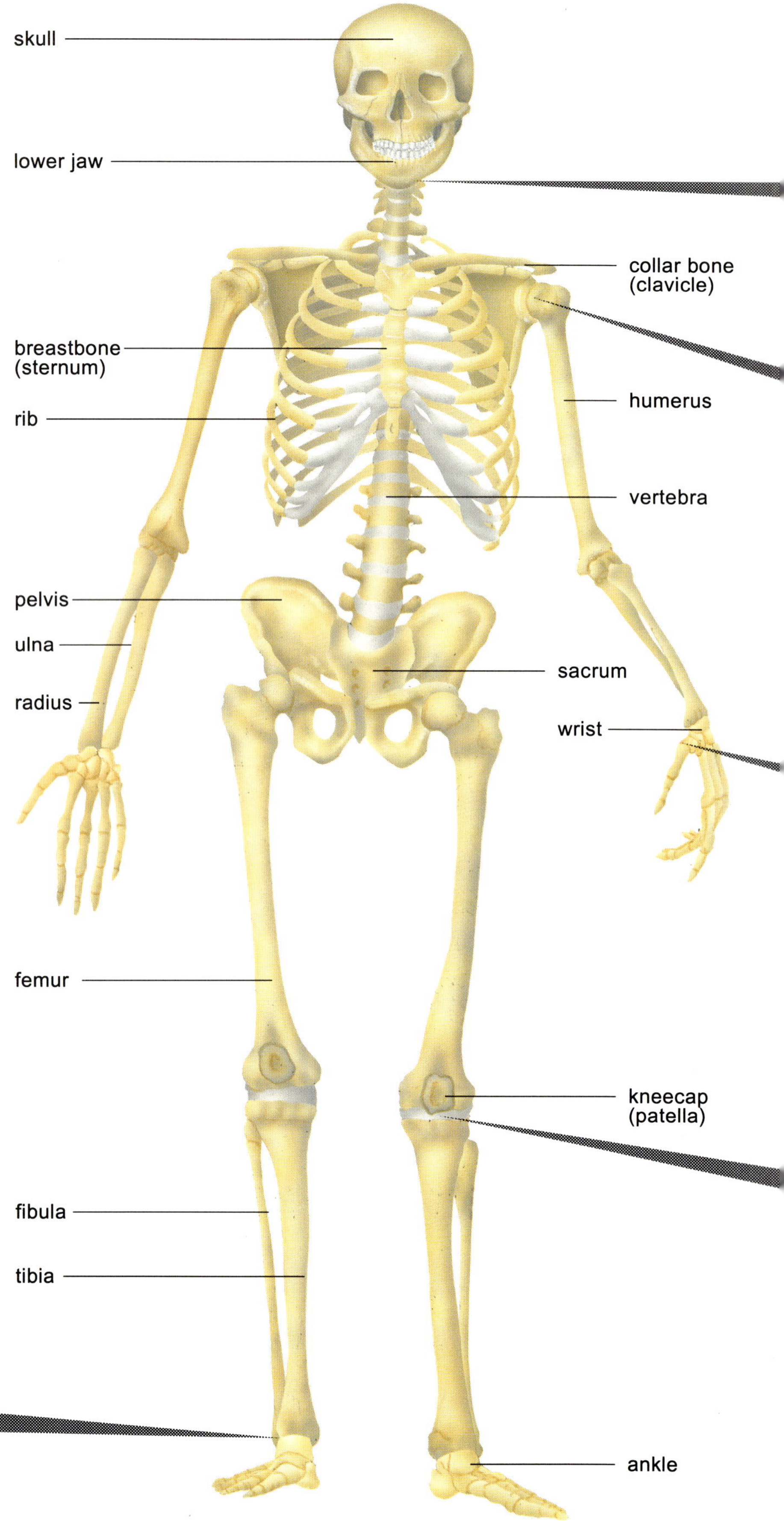

JOINTS

Bones aren't glued together. If they were, you wouldn't be able to move in different directions.

Instead, they have joints. Where the bones meet, they are joined by ligaments: strong sinews (a type of connective tissue). There are five sorts of joints in your body.

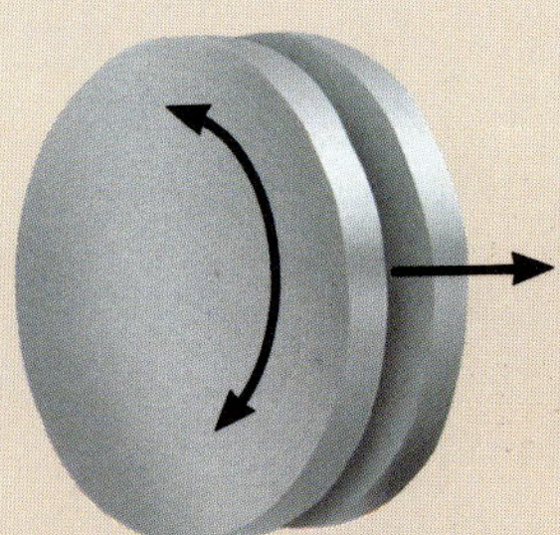

Slipping joints move in many different ways. These joints allow you to do lots of things with your wrists and ankles.

The skull and the spine are joined by a swivel (pivot) joint, so you can turn your head from side to side.

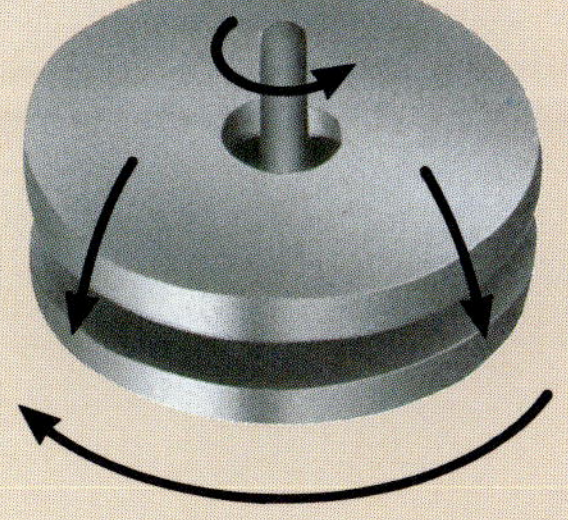

A ball and socket joint allows circular movement. You can swing your arm round because of a ball-and-socket joint at your shoulder. You can circle your leg because of a ball-and-socket joint at your hip.

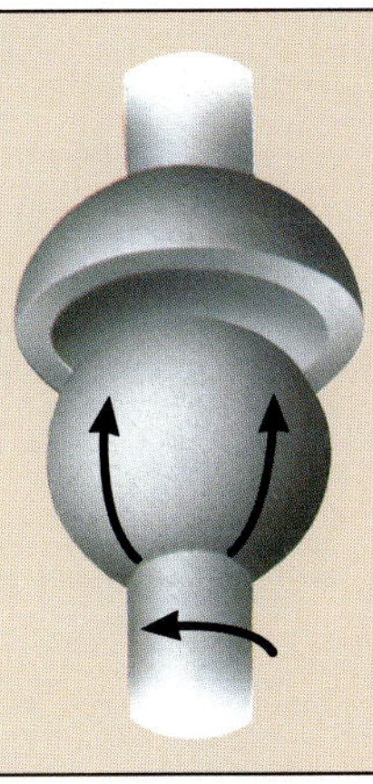

The thumb has a saddle joint which allows up-and-down and side-to-side movements.

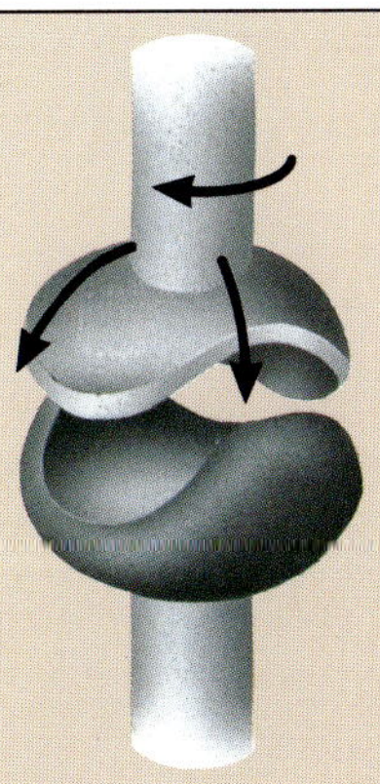

A hinge joint works like a door opening and closing. A hinge joint at the elbow allows you to bend and straighten your arm. Another at the knee allows you to bend and straighten your leg. Your fingers have hinge joints.

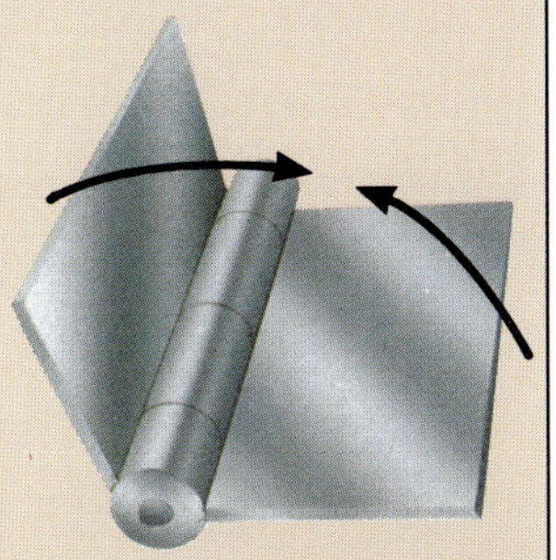

ON THE MEND

Your body is fairly tough and bends easily. But sometimes if you fall awkwardly you break a bone. A child's broken bone usually mends easily. Older people find their bones take longer to heal, and sometimes do not mend very well.

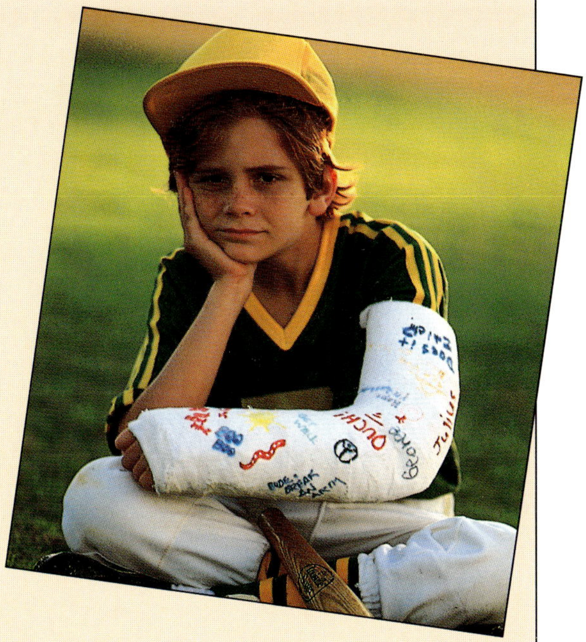

When a bone is broken, the hospital team will often put a bandage stiffened with plaster around it. This plaster cast helps make sure that the bones are held in a line so they mend in the right position. Without the cast they might mend crooked.

How a bone mends

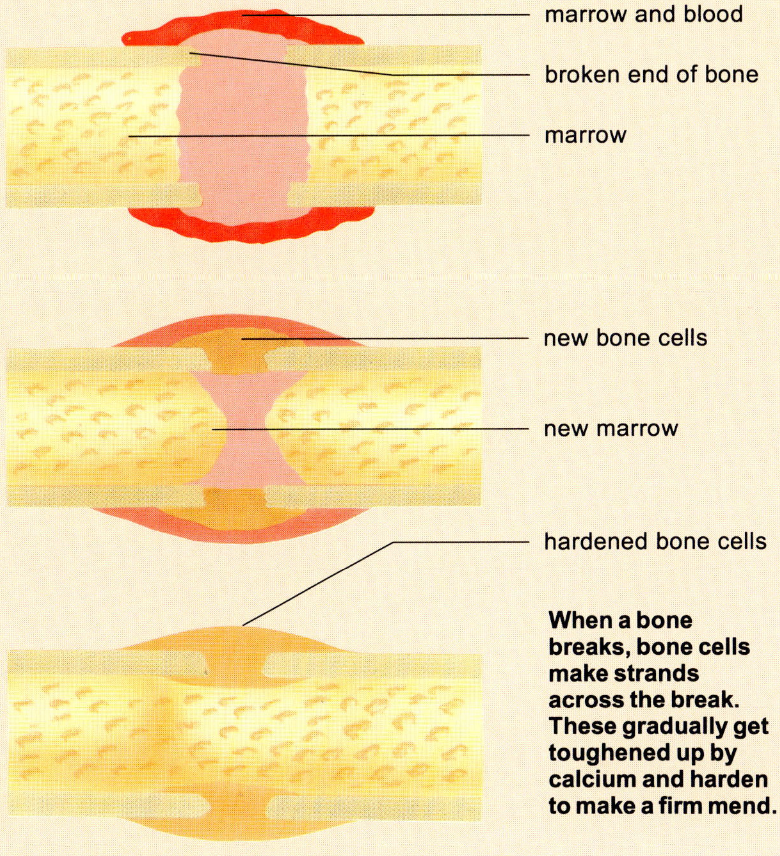

When a bone breaks, bone cells make strands across the break. These gradually get toughened up by calcium and harden to make a firm mend.

MAKING YOU MOVE—MUSCLES

Muscles are the organs that make you move. They are rather like elastic in reverse. Elastic can stretch, and then go back to normal. Muscles can contract—get shorter—and then go back to normal. It's their ability to shorten that makes you move.

Many muscles join on to bones, and cover them. These muscles enable you to move your arms and legs, head and neck . . . and so on. There are lots of other muscles not attached to bones. When you laugh, muscles under the skin of your face ripple with enjoyment, your mouth smiles, your eyes crease up and your tongue curls.

UNDER ORDERS

The thinking part of your brain controls most of your muscles.

When your brain tells you you're late and need to hurry, your brain acts to get your leg muscles moving to make you run, and your arms swinging to help you keep your balance.

There are a few muscles that don't need to wait for special order from the brain. Instead they just keep working. These are special muscles, such as the heart muscle that goes on pumping as long as you are alive, muscles in your intestine that push food downwards through the digestive system, and the muscles that keep you breathing.

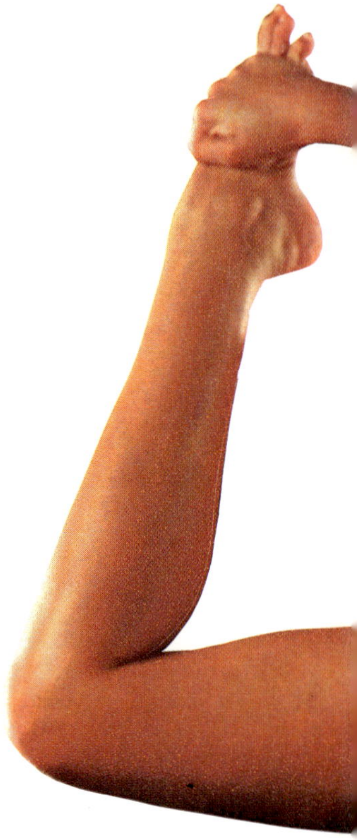

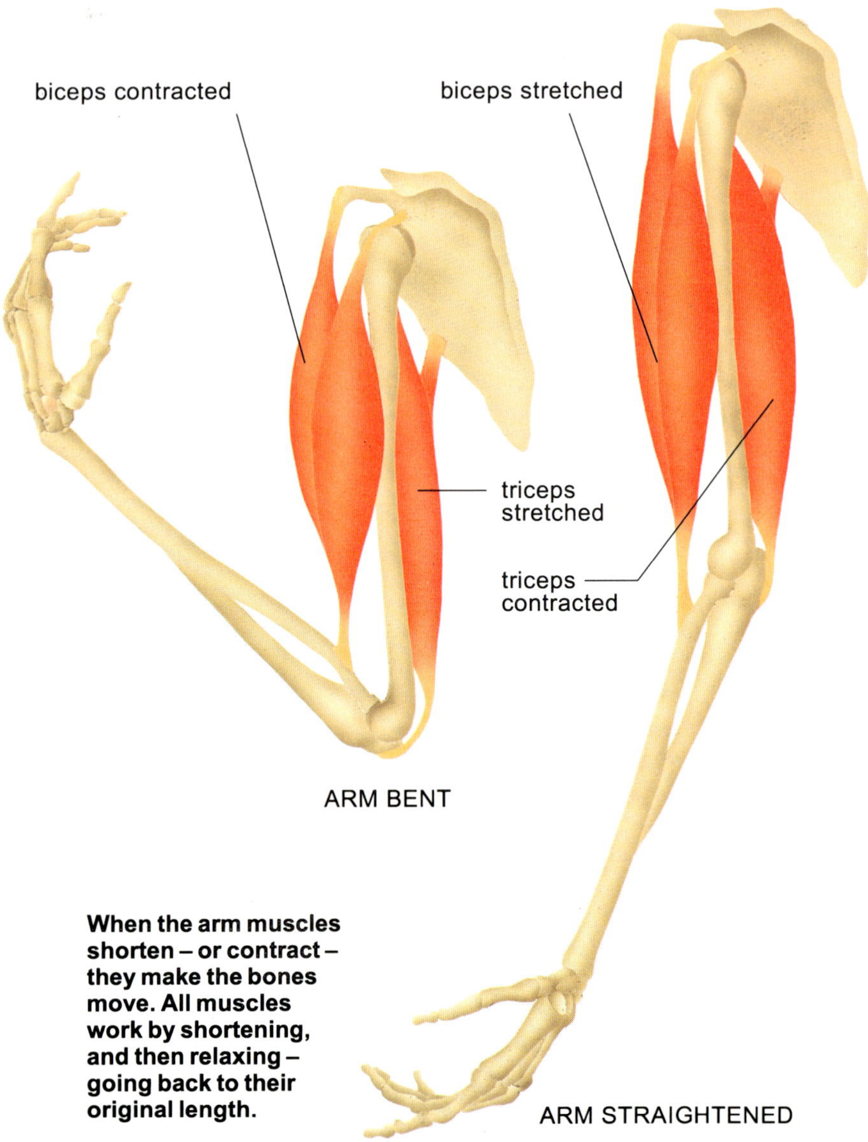

When the arm muscles shorten – or contract – they make the bones move. All muscles work by shortening, and then relaxing – going back to their original length.

DETAILS, DETAILS

When people think of people with well-trained muscles, they often think of people involved in sports, athletics and dance. But trained muscles are also needed for detailed work that requires more skill than strength: embroidery for example, or playing a musical instrument.

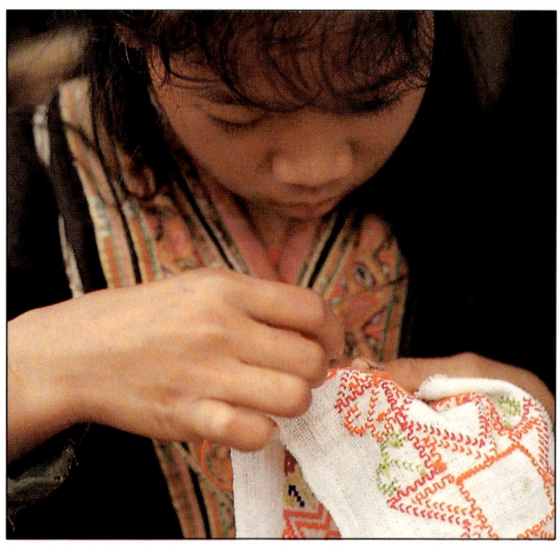

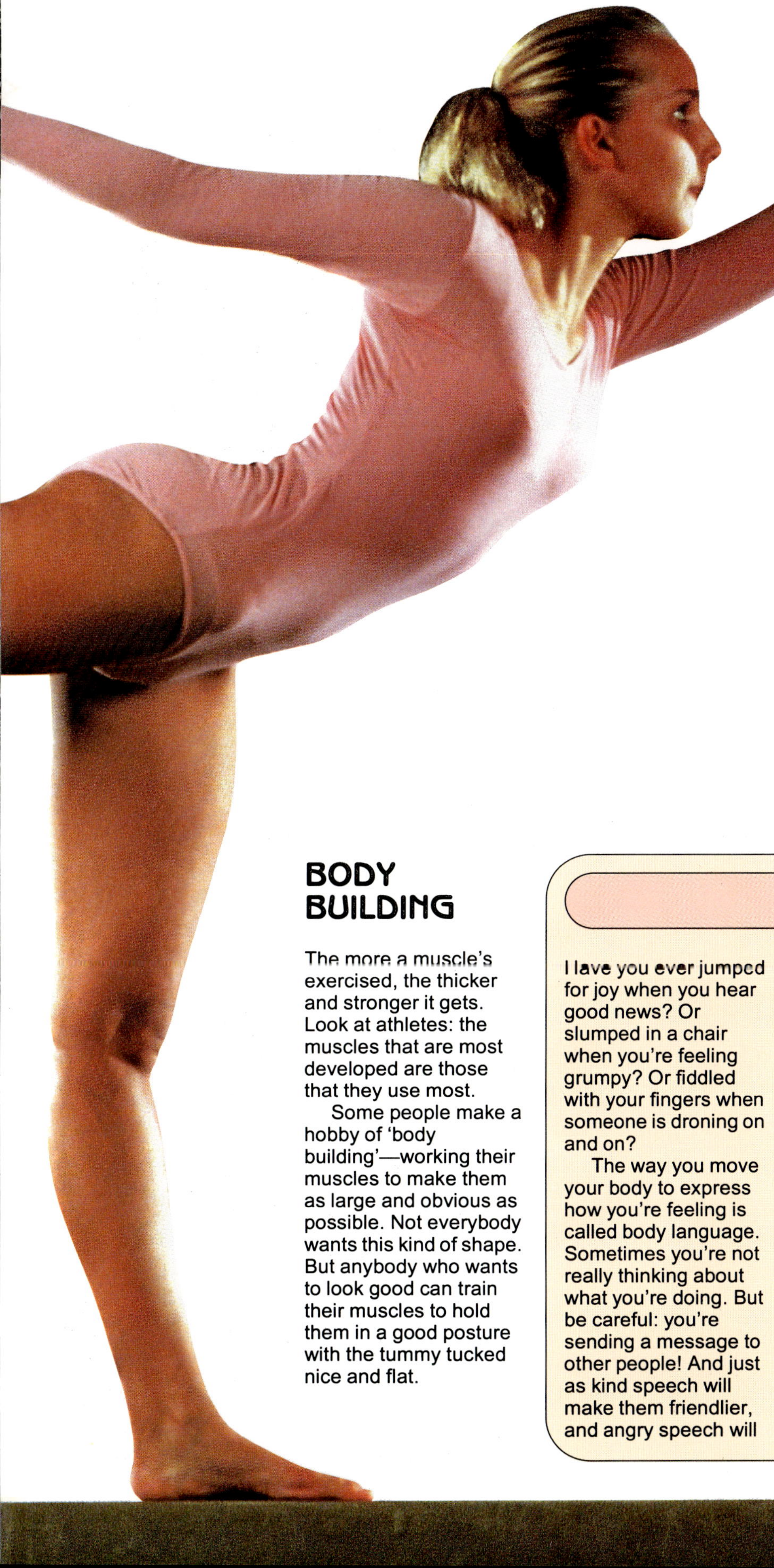

A BALANCED APPROACH

Your body is wonderfully made so that all your muscle movements are balanced carefully. If you do a cartwheel, then the muscles in your arms, legs, stomach wall and back work in harmony to make the cartwheel perfect.

Of course, everything takes practice. A toddler has to practise walking—and takes quite a few tumbles—before the muscles really get the hang of walking. A cartwheel takes lots of practice. Athletics, gymnastics and dance can require even more practice to get the muscle movements just right.

BODY BUILDING

The more a muscle's exercised, the thicker and stronger it gets. Look at athletes: the muscles that are most developed are those that they use most.

Some people make a hobby of 'body building'—working their muscles to make them as large and obvious as possible. Not everybody wants this kind of shape. But anybody who wants to look good can train their muscles to hold them in a good posture with the tummy tucked nice and flat.

BODY TALK

Have you ever jumped for joy when you hear good news? Or slumped in a chair when you're feeling grumpy? Or fiddled with your fingers when someone is droning on and on?

The way you move your body to express how you're feeling is called body language. Sometimes you're not really thinking about what you're doing. But be careful: you're sending a message to other people! And just as kind speech will make them friendlier, and angry speech will make them angrier, body messages will affect the way they deal with you.

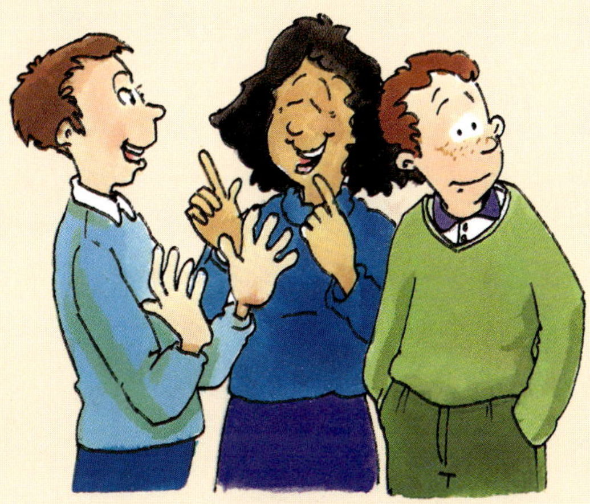

WHAT'S THE POINT?

Bodies go through lots of different stages. A baby grows into a child, then into a teenager, and eventually into an adult. By that stage, growing is complete.

The body continues to renew and repair itself, but as the years go by, other changes take place. Hair changes colour, the skin may begin to sag a little, and wrinkle. Sight and hearing may be less good. Bones become more fragile . . . the body is wearing out.

At some stage, everyone has to die. Many people die simply when their bodies are old and worn out. Others die of illnesses that stop their body working, or accidents that damage the body.

When a person is dead, the heart stops beating, the brain stops dealing with messages, and the body stops working. It will be buried or cremated.

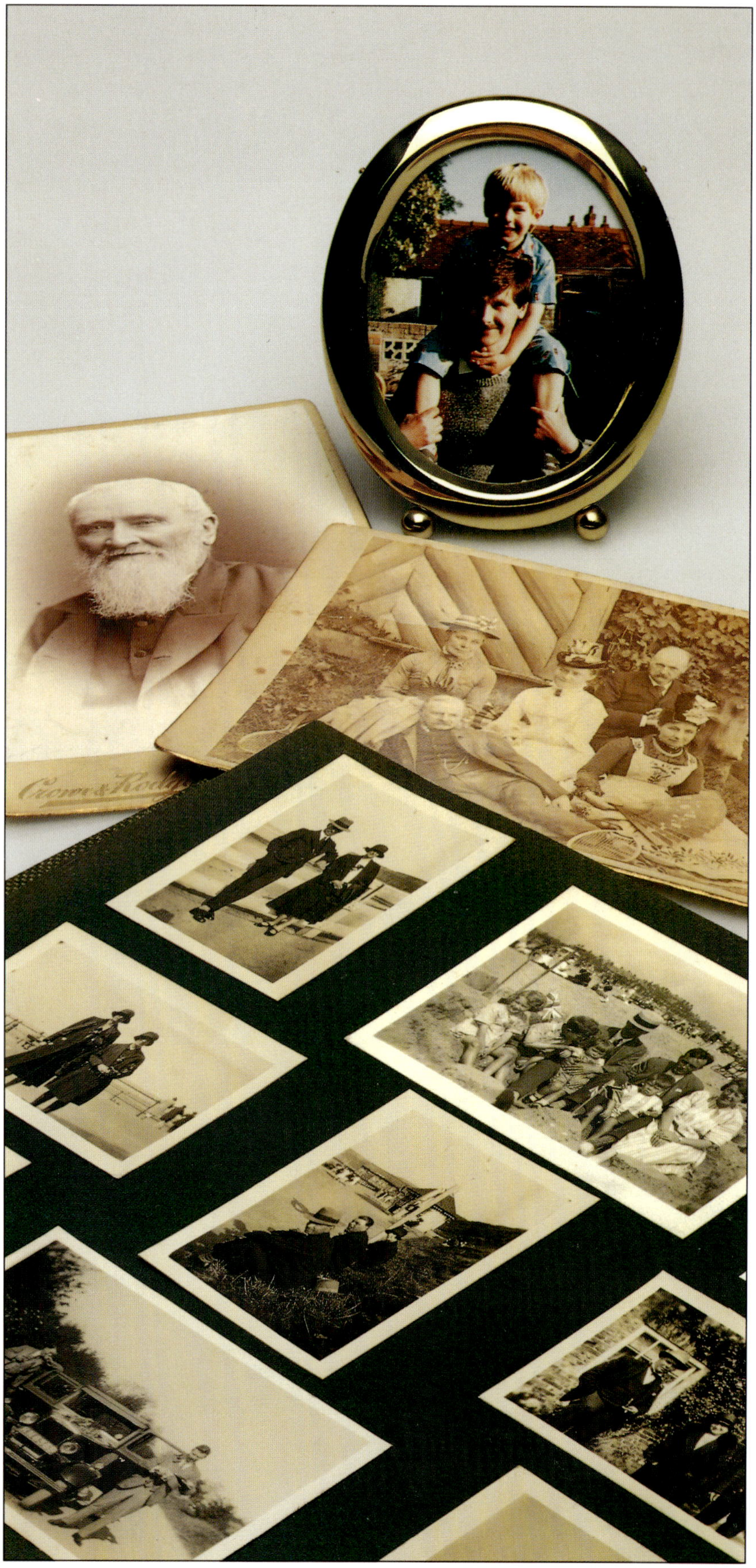

WHAT HAPPENS AFTER DEATH?

Scientists can't track anything that has escaped from the body when it dies, but without the life inside, the person has gone. What has happened to that?

People from different backgrounds have many different ideas about what happens after death. For example, the Bible that Jews and Christians share (as well as the Muslim Qur'an) explains that at death people move on to a different type of existence. This is called 'eternal life', and it brings them face to face with the God who, they believe, made the world, and loves the people in it.

The Christian Bible includes stories about a person named Jesus who was put to death by his enemies in spite of a lifetime spent showing people the good and right way to live. Christians believe that Jesus was God's son: because God's son suffered a cruel death as a human being, they believe that God really understands the grief caused by death.

The stories of Jesus also include reports of people who claimed to have seen Jesus alive again after he had been killed. This gives Christians a special reason for believing that there is life after death.

WHAT NOW?

It's amazing what you can do with your body. What you do with your body—and the mind inside it—affects what you do with your life. Will you be good at making things? Or good at sports? Perhaps you are specially good at making friends with people, and helping them to laugh and have a good time.

There are lots and lots of choices about what to do with the life you have. And although adults may help decide what you do now, as you grow up you're going to start making the decisions.

So it's worth thinking hard about how you're going to answer some of the questions you'll face. Questions such as how to treat other people, what to spend your time doing, how to treat the world around you. Is there a 'right' way to behave?

Your life is not just about taking care of your body: it's about using every part of you in a good way.

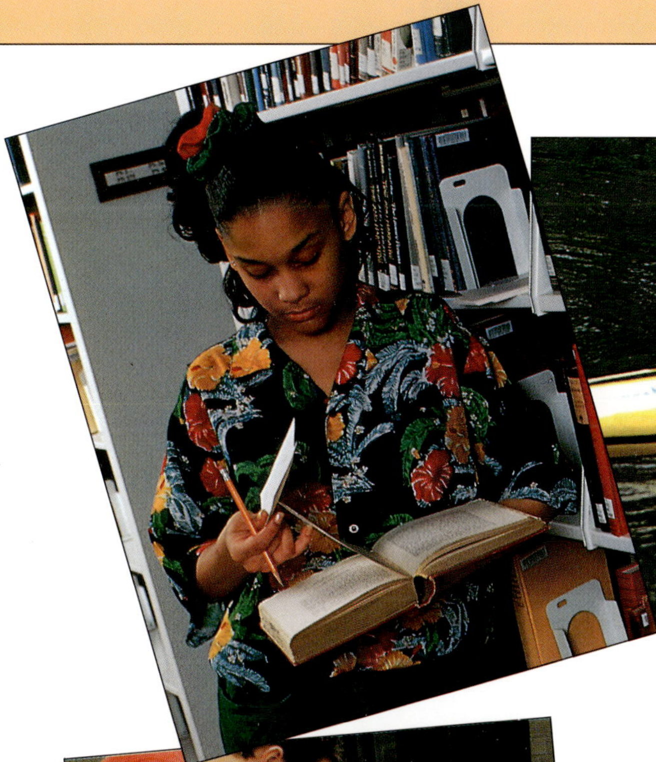

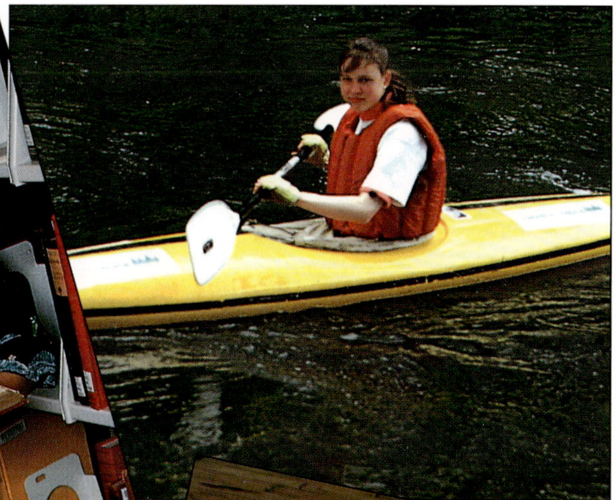

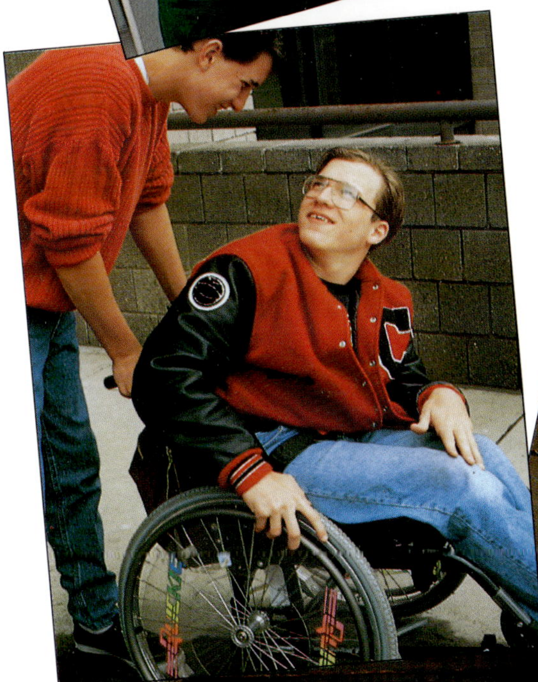

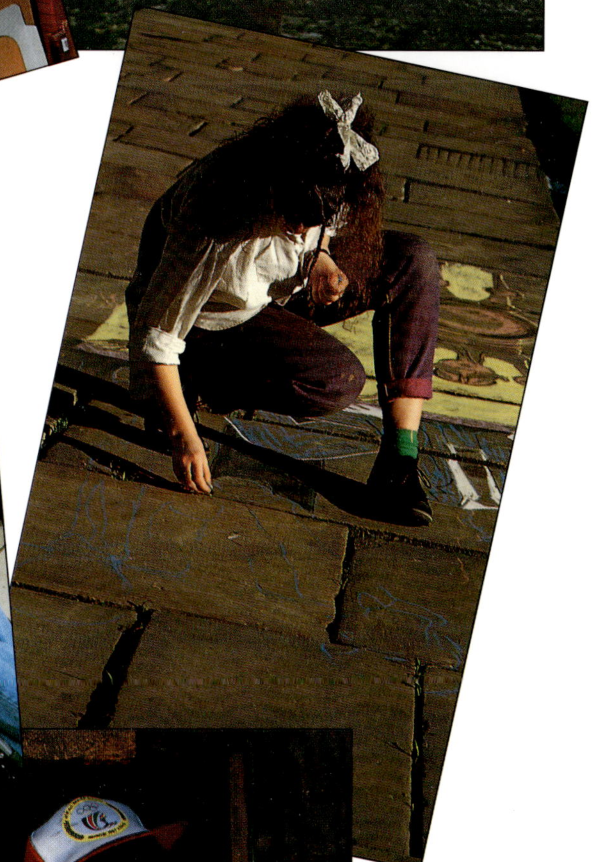

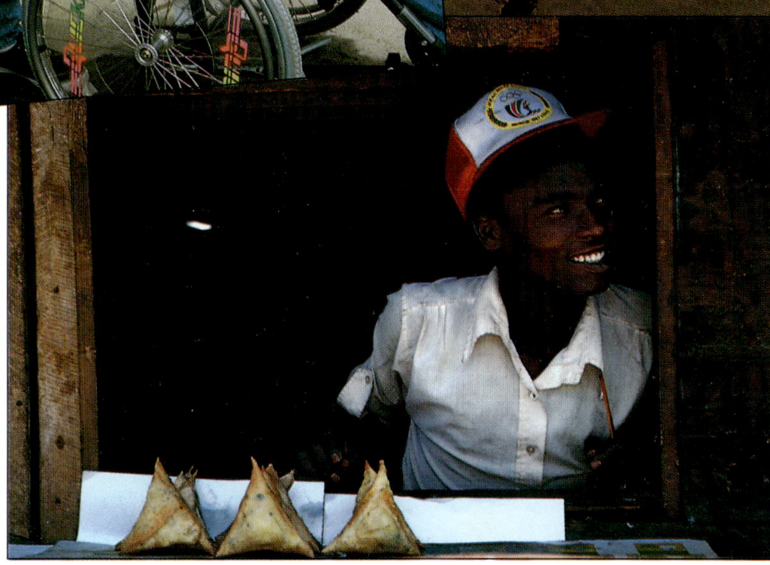

What will you do with your life? The choices you make as you grow up will affect what you do as an adult.

INDEX